Medicare For All

Healthcare continues to be one of the defining political issues in the United States. Though many progressives argue for an overhaul of the current system based on ethical or humanitarian principles, this important book offers an economic rationale for providing healthcare for all.

The purpose of *Medicare For All: An Economic Rationale* is to demonstrate how current runaway healthcare prices can be addressed by implementing the cost-effectiveness of Medicare For All. Written by a former Corporate Director and healthcare consultant, this book illustrates why the current free market model for healthcare is ultimately failing the country by not containing rising healthcare costs, which has a severe economic impact on all Americans, including those covered by employer medical plans. Major factors in that failure such as the lack of transparency, human decision factors, and high administrative costs in the current system are explored. The book demonstrates that implementing Medicare For All, providing comprehensive benefits with no copays, private insurance premiums, deductibles, or other cost-sharing, will not only improve the lives of most Americans, but will be far more cost-effective than the present system.

This is an incisive, important contribution to a topic that continues to shape American political discourse and will be of interest to scholars and professionals engaged in this area as well as politicians and the public in general.

Ken Lefkowitz is a former consultant and Senior Director for major corporations, including AstraZeneca and PECO Energy. Ken designed and managed healthcare plans for hundreds of thousands of employees and their dependents. He has negotiated with major health insurers and managed large corporate self-insured plans. A number of his writings about healthcare have been published in the *Washington Post*, *Courier Post/USA Today Network*, *Philadelphia Inquirer*, and the *New York Times*. Ken earned a BA degree from Brooklyn College, MS degree from City University of NY, and pursued graduate business studies at St. Johns University.

Medicare For All
An Economic Rationale

Ken Lefkowitz

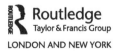 Routledge
Taylor & Francis Group

LONDON AND NEW YORK

First published 2022
by Routledge
4 Park Square, Milton Park, Abingdon, Oxon OX14 4RN

and by Routledge
605 Third Avenue, New York, NY 10158

Routledge is an imprint of the Taylor & Francis Group, an informa business

© 2022 Ken Lefkowitz

British Library Cataloguing-in-Publication Data
A catalogue record for this book is available from the British Library

Library of Congress Cataloging-in-Publication Data
A catalog record has been requested for this book

ISBN: 978-1-032-22341-4 (hbk)
ISBN: 978-1-032-26049-5 (pbk)
ISBN: 978-1-003-28627-1 (ebk)

DOI: 10.4324/9781003286271

Typeset in Times New Roman
by codeMantra

Contents

Figures

Tables

Acknowledgments

Many thanks to Dr. Lisa Taylor, PhD and Dr. Dan Lefkowitz, PhD for their questions and challenges which helped sharpen the focus and positions in this book. Further thanks to Dr. Lefkowitz for his many hours of help and support in proofing and testing formats of the book to meet scholarly, academic, and publishing standards. His help and contributions were invaluable.

The author extends his deep appreciation to the organization PNHP, Physicians for a National Health Program, a major advocacy organization for Medicare For All. The information, research, guidance, presentations, and articles written by their members, and shared on their website for all members, have been invaluable in the writing of this book. They have been posting the articles/letters of mine that have appeared in *The New York Times*, *Philadelphia Inquirer*, and *Washington Post* about Medicare For All on their website. May I thank them for that too, especially Communications Specialist, Clare Fauke.

May I extend a warm thank you to Mr. Ralph Hendrickson, head of the Steering Committee of the organization SJNOWIndivisible which he leads with great skill, and on which I serve. After a presentation he invited me to make to the group, Ralph provided me the encouragement, inspiration, and motivation to complete "Medicare For All: An Economic Rationale."

1 A Brief Background and Outline of the Book

Background/Overview

Healthcare has been at the forefront of critical issues in America for the past decade and continues to preoccupy the public conscience. The passage of the Affordable Care Act in 2010 clearly solidified healthcare as a major focus of the national political debate. The loss of coverage associated with the COVID-19 pandemic, media emphasis on surprise billing, and the expansion of the Affordable Care Act as part of the recently passed stimulus bill focuses even more attention on the subject. Additionally, the reintroduction of Medicare For All in the House of Representatives by Congresswoman Pramila Jayapal on March 21, 2021, and similar action expected to follow in the Senate by Bernie Sanders, ensures healthcare will continue to be among the nation's preeminent issues.

Any consideration of healthcare must, by definition, include the concept of Medicare For All, introduced to the American public by its champion and major sponsor Senator Bernie Sanders, especially during the Democratic Presidential debates leading up to the 2020 presidential election. Senator Sanders' emphasis on healthcare as a human right, the inequality of our current healthcare system, and the excesses of the insurance industry represent his leading themes in proposing Medicare For All, becoming rallying cries for its progressive and liberal supporters.

These themes were recently echoed again on March 17, 2021, when US Congresswoman Pramila Jayapal, representing Washington State's 7th District, and Congresswoman Debbie Dingell, representing Michigan's 12th District in the US House of Representatives, introduced the Medicare For All Act of 2021. This legislation would guarantee healthcare to everyone in America providing comprehensive benefits with no co-pays, private insurance premiums, deductibles, or other cost-sharing. Many speakers participated during their "town hall" meeting, explaining why they supported Medicare For All, including the heads of organizations championing the bill as well as other prominent members of the Democratic Party. Some emphasis was placed on the pandemic and how unemployment skyrocketed to historic levels, causing millions of

DOI: 10.4324/9781003286271-1

Americans to lose their health insurance. However, the speakers' focus was on Senator Sanders' themes already repeated numerous times emphasizing social, humanitarian, ethical, and equality issues. Healthcare as a human right, patients over profits, and the plight of uninsured and underinsured Americans were consistently repeated. And that is to be expected since the essence of the system is to expand comprehensive first dollar healthcare coverage to every citizen. Therefore, emphasis has been on healthcare as a human right, eliminating the uninsured and underinsured, while addressing racial and economic inequities.

Although these issues are certainly quite important and highly relevant, they fall short of presenting the entire picture. It is the purpose of this book to complete the key missing piece: current runaway healthcare prices versus the cost-effectiveness of Medicare For All. In order to accomplish this, we will first explore the high cost of our current free market system and its dismal and continuing failure to control healthcare costs. As major factors in that failure, we will explain the lack of transparency and the human decision factors in the current system, as well as its high administrative costs. Then, in contrast to the free market system, we will demonstrate the cost-effectiveness of Medicare For All.

Progressives and Democrats would be better served by shifting their focus to gain additional support among moderates and even some cost-minded conservatives. Emphasizing why our broken free market system has failed dismally in controlling costs, allowing runaway healthcare costs to continue, affecting all Americans, and then demonstrating how these costs can be contained is an approach that should garner broader support. Warren Buffet, the renowned investor and Chief Executive Officer of Berkshire Hathaway, was quoted as saying that ballooning medical costs are, "A hungry tapeworm on the American Economy."[1] Demonstrating how the American economy overall and every individual's economic situation is eroded by runaway healthcare costs, using a "follow the money" approach, would surely gain increased and even perhaps strong support for Medicare For All, moving beyond progressive and liberal ranks to many more American citizens of all political persuasions and value systems. That is the purpose of "Medicare For All: An Economic Rationale."

Outline of Medicare For All

Before we begin the exploration of our current system's flaws and shortcomings, it is important to outline the definition of Medicare For All so the reader can gain an understanding of the program's essentials and parameters. Two Medicare For All bills have been introduced in Congress, one originally in the House by Representative Jayapal, HR 1384 in March 2019, and another in the Senate, S1129, by Senator Sanders in April 2019, who humorously said in a discussion about Medicare For

All elements during the Democratic Presidential debates, "I wrote the damn bill." Quite similar in content, both bills present the key elements of a Medicare For All program, defining it as a single-payer universal healthcare coverage plan. Here are their key elements:

- Every resident receives a healthcare coverage card;
- Comprehensive coverage is provided for doctor, hospital, dental, vision, mental health, medical supplies, pharmaceuticals, and long-term care;
- There are no deductibles or copays;
- Private duplicate coverage is banned;
- The plans are exempt from the Hyde Amendment that bans government spending on women's right to choose.

Under each plan, doctors, hospitals, and other medical providers remain independent and operate freely. Patients are free to choose any doctor or hospital since the delivery of care continues to remain in private hands. Continued free choice of each person to select their own doctors and hospitals is assured. Neither plan is a government takeover of healthcare. Only funding and coverage are addressed.

Reference List

1 "A Good Health Care Deal, But Only for Some," by Elisabeth Rosenthal, *NY Times*, Feb 1, 2018, https://www.nytimes.com/2018/02/02/opinion/health-care-berkshire-amazon-chase.html.

2   America's Healthcare Costs and Quality

America spent $3.8 trillion on healthcare in 2019. That accounted for 17.7% of gross domestic product (GDP) and has been increasing nearly every year for the past few decades. The amount is alarming and as mentioned in the prior chapter, Warren Buffet, the renowned investor and Chief Executive Officer of Berkshire Hathaway, was quoted as saying that ballooning medical costs are, "A hungry tapeworm on the American Economy."[1] A most visually disturbing image as can be imagined.

Although in absolute terms the $3.8 billion is a staggering sum, expenditures on healthcare when compared with other countries are even more pronounced and concerning.

Figure 2.1 presents US spending when compared to other highly industrialized advanced countries. The spending data are expressed as dollars per capita per year. The major source of the data is the Organisation for Economic Co-operation and Development, OECD, which is an intergovernmental economic organization with 37 member countries respected

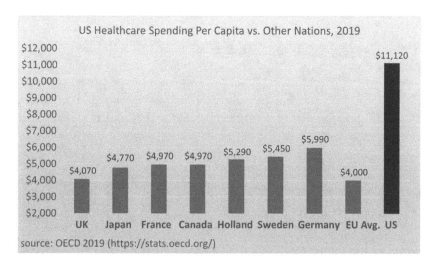

Figure 2.1 US Healthcare Spending Per Capita versus Other Nations, 2019

DOI: 10.4324/9781003286271-2

for its studies of comparative economic data and evaluations of its member nations.[2]

The UK spends the least at about $4,000 followed by Japan, France, Canada, Holland, and Sweden clustered around $5,000. Germany is next at closer to $6,000. For a broader perspective, we calculated the average of the European Union which is very nearly the same as the UK at $4,000. The most striking amount on the chart is the United States that spends in excess of $11,000, more than twice that of all the other countries except one. That country is Germany against whom the United States falls just short of spending double.

It is important to note that many types of healthcare systems are represented in the chart above. For instance, the UK has nationalized health insurance while Canada uses a single-payer system that is funded through the national government and administered by the Provinces, which are roughly equivalent to states in America. The Canadian healthcare system is financed with general revenue raised through federal, provincial, and territorial taxation. Physicians, hospitals, and other healthcare providers are independent and free to practice as they chose. We will be referring to the Canadian single-payer system numerous times throughout this book, and therefore, a more detailed description of the system is provided in the Appendix.

Germany is an example of other healthcare systems. Universal health insurance is mandatory and is a mix of funding systems. First is the statutory health insurance system, or SHI, consisting of sickness funds. These are not-for-profit, competing, non-government health insurance plans. Sickness funds are financed by employers and workers through general wage contributions. Second is private health insurance. The federal government has wide-ranging regulatory power over healthcare but is not directly involved in care delivery. The Federal Joint Committee, supervised by the Federal Ministry of Health, determines the services to be covered by sickness funds. A key point is that the government has the responsibility and control over setting prices. The government plays a strong controlling role in private health insurance. It is regulated by the Ministry of Health and the Federal Financial Supervisory Authority in many ways including premium increases. This is a limited general outline of the German system, and because it is a system that has private health insurance and that is heavily controlled by the government, including pricing, a more detailed description is provided in the Appendix.

The rather dramatic difference in spending between the United States and other countries as shown in Figure 2.1 may easily lead us to believe that the quality and performance of healthcare in the United States is at a level far in advance of other nations. However, most alarming is the fact that despite the high cost, the United States was ranked last of 11 developed countries in performance and quality by the Commonwealth Fund Study of Health Quality.[3] Such a contrast is not just disturbing from an overall health perspective, it also indicates quite clearly that our country is failing miserably in getting value for its healthcare dollar. An analogy is a person who paid $1,000 for a service they could purchase elsewhere for $512. We all would consider such a person quite foolish. Yet, that's the situation facing healthcare in America today.

The charts on the following pages clearly display categories in which the United States sadly lags behind other countries.

First is Life Expectancy, a generally accepted measure of healthcare quality as shown in Figure 2.2. Of course, quite a few other factors are involved in life span, but healthcare is a major determinant. The Life Expectancy Chart clearly demonstrates that the United States trails other industrialized countries at 78.6 years compared with Germany, the UK, Canada, France, Sweden, and Italy in which citizens live between 81 and 83 years.

Another quality measure is Infant Mortality. As Figure 2.3 clearly shows, the United States tragically leads most industrialized nations. The United States has 5.9 deaths in the first year of life per 1,000 births, compared with Canada at 4.5, France at 3.8, Germany and Australia at 3.3, Italy at 2.7, and Sweden at the lowest of 2.4 deaths per 1,000 births in the first year of life.

A third important quality measure is maternal mortality, expressed as deaths per 100,000 births. Here, again, as can be clearly seen on Figure 2.4, the United States has a dismal record when compared with other industrialized countries. The United States leads the pack by far with an appalling 26.4 maternal deaths per 100,000 births compared with France, Canada, the UK, Germany, and Australia which ranged from a low of 1.6 deaths to 8.7 deaths.

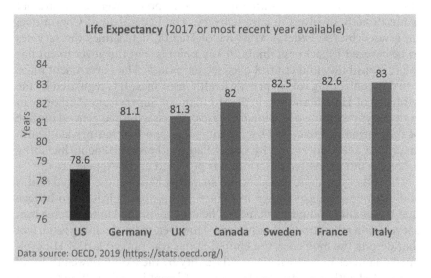

Figure 2.2 A comparison of life expectancy in the United States versus other countries

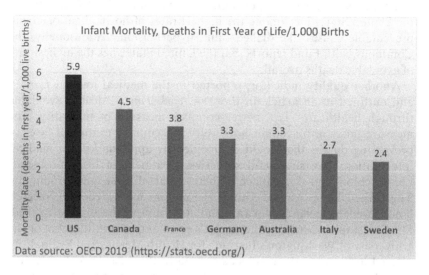

Figure 2.3 A comparison of infant mortality in the United States versus other countries

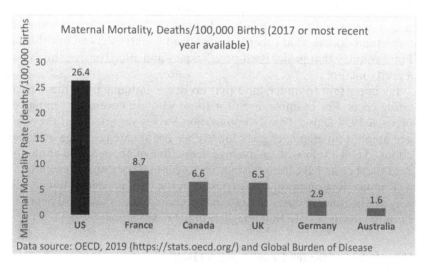

Figure 2.4 A comparison of maternal mortality in the United States versus other countries

In addition to these three measures focusing on longevity, a number of studies including those reported by the Commonwealth Fund indicate that the United States also performs poorly in managing chronic disease, which in its many forms is growing in America.[3] Chronic disease includes arthritis, asthma, chronic lung disease, diabetes, heart disease, heart attack, hypertension, or high blood pressure. The OECD reports the United States has among the highest rates of hospitalizations from preventable causes like diabetes and hypertension.[2] Additionally, the Commonwealth Fund reports that the United States has the highest rate of avoidable deaths overall.[3]

Another quality indicator, reported in the medical journal *Lancet*, and outlined in an article in the *New York Times*, "deaths avoidable through healthcare" is a newer complex measure of mortality. The measure takes into account how well each country examined fares at preventing deaths that could be avoided by applying known medical interventions like successful surgeries, treatment of birth problems, breast, colon, and skin cancer, diabetes, heart disease, and lymphoma. The United States ranked 35th of the nations measured with Switzerland, Sweden, Iceland, Norway, and Australia at the highest ranked. Dr. Christopher Murphy, the report's chief author and director of the University of Washington's Institute for Health Metrics and Evaluation, offered his view of the results as quoted in the *New York Times*, "It's an embarrassment, especially considering how much the US spends on healthcare per person."[4]

Dr. Murphy's comment sums up the key point of this chapter, compared with other countries, the quality of healthcare in the United States is far from exemplary, especially in light of the fact that America spends more than double what other industrialized countries do on healthcare. For a country that prides itself on efficiency and effectiveness, this is not a pretty picture.

It's important to understand that no one is immune from these escalating costs. For example, even for those who are covered by employer plans, a 2020 Kaiser Family Foundation Survey reported that the average amount an employee pays for his/her healthcare coverage averages about $5,600 a year with an average deductible of about $1,650 annually. And these costs have been raising every year and continue to escalate.[5]

The puzzling question that arises from the data presented thus far is, why are healthcare costs so high in the United States? We will begin to examine the answer to that question in the next section.

Why US Healthcare Costs Are So High?

In the previous section, we explored the costs of US healthcare and examined them in the light of the low return on healthcare dollars as measured by quality. That examination begs the question: Why are our costs so high?

There can be a number of reasons including bad health habits, age of the population, and the overuse of care. We'll examine each of these factors.

Figures 2.5, 2.6, and 2.7 present an overview of the US population compared to other countries. First is the prevalence of smoking, a major cause of lung disease, cancer, cardiovascular illness, and short-ened life span. Figure 2.5 presents the percent of the countries' popu-lation older than 15 who are smokers. The United States is nearly tied with Sweden for the lowest percentage at 10.5% and 10.4%, respectively. Canada, Australia, the UK, Italy, and France all have substantially higher rates of smokers in their population, with France the highest at 22.9%. So, clearly, smoking is not a factor in America's high health-care cost when compared with other countries. In fact, based on the habit of smoking, a major cause of disease, with all other factors being the same, the United States should have lower healthcare costs. It is important to recognize that we are generalizing here from smoking as representing more healthy lifestyles. Another element affecting health is obesity where the United States ranks higher against other countries than smoking

In Figure 2.6, the next factor we will examine that can drive healthcare costs upward is the age of the population. As people age, the cost of their healthcare cost rises with the greater incidence of disease, illness, and the increasing need for care.

Here, as with the prevalence of smoking, the United Stated compares favorably with other industrialized nations. In fact, the US percent of population 65 years of age and older is the lowest among the comparison group of countries at 16%. The percentage of senior citizens in the popu-lations of Canada, the UK, France, Sweden, Germany, Italy, and Japan ranges from 17.3% in Canada to a high of 28.2% in Japan, all substantially greater than the United States. We would expect the lower percentage of

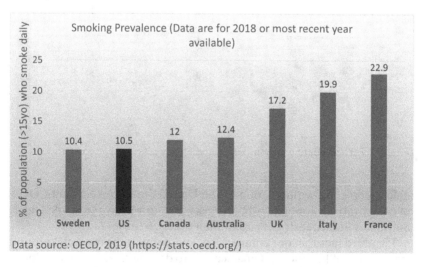

Figure 2.5 Smoking prevalence in the United States versus other countries

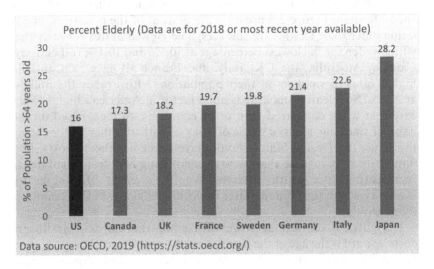

Figure 2.6 Percent elderly in the United States versus other countries

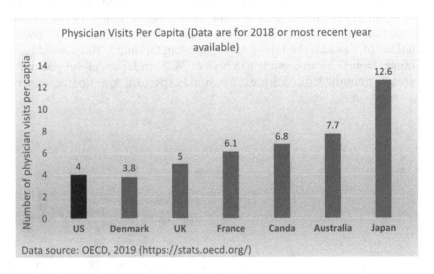

Figure 2.7 Healthcare usage in the United States versus other countries

older people in the population of the United States to be a major factor in comparatively lower healthcare costs. Yet, as we have seen, the United States has higher costs per capita than other countries.

The third factor in our comparison, and perhaps the most meaningful, is the usage of healthcare. One measure to determine this usage is doctor visits per capita as shown in Figure 2.7.

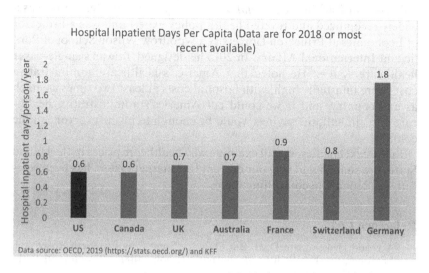

Figure 2.8 Hospital inpatient days per capita

The United States has next to the lowest number of visits to a doctor at 4.0 a year. Denmark is lower, but nearly the same at 3.8. The other countries, the UK, France, Canada, Australia, and Japan, all are higher ranging from 5.0 visits per year in the UK to 12.6 in Japan.

Another helpful measure of usage is hospital stays as indicated by Hospital Inpatient Days Per Capita in Figure 2.8.

In addition to the OECD, the Kaiser Family Foundation, KFF, is the source of the data. KFF is a widely known and trusted source of facts, polling, and analysis focused on healthcare issues and policy.[5]

The United States has the lowest inpatient days per person at 0.6 per year, the same as Canada. The UK, Australia, France, Switzerland, and Germany all have higher hospital usage ranging from 0.7 in the UK to 1.8 inpatient days per person per year.

This examination shows that the United States population's use of healthcare gauged by doctor visits and hospital stays is low when compared with other industrialized nations, eliminating usage as a factor in the high level of US healthcare costs.

So, if high healthcare costs in America don't result from poor health habits, older age of the population, or overuse of care, then what is the cause of our extremely high healthcare costs?

"It's the Prices, Stupid"

This was the explanation provided publicly and in speeches and seminars by recently deceased Professor Uwe Reinhardt based on a study published in 2003 in the *Journal of Health Affairs.*[6] Dr. Reinhardt was a widely recognized and revered health policy expert and was a Professor of Economics at Princeton University's Woodrow Wilson School of Public and International Affairs. In 2015 he designed Taiwan's single-payer healthcare system. He noted that America's healthcare administrative costs were unusually high, with hospital costs at least two times as much as any country, and if we could cut America's administrative healthcare costs in half, the savings would be enough to insure everyone in the country.

In the next chapter we will examine why healthcare prices in the United States are so high and why our current free market system has been woefully inadequate in controlling them.

Reference List

1 "A Good Health Care Deal, But Only for Some," by Elisabeth Rosenthal, *NY Times*, Feb 1, 2018, https://www.nytimes.com/2018/02/02/opinion/healthcare-berkshire-amazon-chase.html.
2 Health Expenditure and Financing, Health Status, OECD, OECD.Stat, https://stats.oecd.org/Index.aspx?DataSetCode=SHA.
3 Health Care in the U.S. Compared to Other High-Income Countries, The Commonwealth Fund, Aug 4, 2021, https://www.commonwealthfund.org/publications/fund-reports/2021/aug/mirror-mirror-2021-reflecting-poorly.
4 Global Health, A Global Scorecard Finds U.S. Lacking, *New York Times*, May 23, 2017, Page D6, https://www.nytimes.com/2017/05/22/health/healthcare-global-united-states.html?searchResultPosition=1.
5 Kaiser Family Foundation 2020 Employer Health Benefits Survey, Published: Oct 8, 2020, https://www.kff.org/health-costs/report/2020-employer-health-benefits-survey/.
6 It's the Prices, Stupid: Why the United States Is So Different from Other Countries, Gerald F. Anderson, Uwe E. Reinhardt, Peter S. Hussey, and Varduhi Petrosyan, *Health Affairs*, 22(3), May/June 2003, https://www.healthaffairs.org/doi/full/10.1377/hlthaff.22.3.89.

3   High Prices and the Free Market System

In the prior chapter we explained the reason for the high costs of health-care in America; As Professor Uwe Reinhardt's research demonstrated, "It's the prices, stupid." Of course, that statement raises the question: so, why are the prices so high? Which is the topic of this current chapter.

Four key factors drive the high healthcare prices in the United States. First is the lack of transparency in our broken free market system. Second is human nature as it relates to the need for healthcare. Third is insurance company administrative and overhead costs which add decision layers, but no value. Fourth is hospital, doctor, and other healthcare provider fees which are driven upward by the third factor, high administrative costs. We will examine each of these factors in this and the next chapter.

Our current American healthcare is financed through a free market. In a free market system, prices are controlled through the process of buyers comparing the price, and quality, of competing products. This process requires transparency so that consumers can make informed choices when they purchase a product or service. Think of a few gas stations operating in the same town within a short drive of each other, a fairly common occurrence in America. Consumers can easily compare prices by reading the posted amounts above the gas pumps or the typically large price signs at each station. Since they have experienced the gasoline sold by each station being relatively the same in quality, consumers can easily compare the price charged and make an informed decision about which gas to buy, gravitating toward the stations offering the lowest prices. Each station is quite aware of the prices charged by the other stations when they set their prices. They may consider other factors such as a more convenient location, but the dominant factor is the price other purveyors charge. Clearly, if one station decides to lower its prices and consumers respond by purchasing from that station, the other stations will be pressured to adjust their prices. And if an additional gas station opens, the other stations will be forced to react to its price as well as the additional supply of gasoline. From the demand side, if consumers decide that gasoline prices are too high, they can cut back on their driving and/or consider using mass transit like buses and trains. The resulting pressure of reduced demand will

DOI: 10.4324/9781003286271-3

over time, barring other factors like the price the stations pay distribu-
tors for gasoline, cause the gas stations to lower their prices.

The above gas station scenario outlines transparency in action and
how it controls pricing within a free market. We can see that transparency
allows the market to determine the price of goods and services through
supply and demand which reflects individual consumer choice through
comparing prices and quality.

An appreciation of transparency and its critical role in free market pricing is important in understanding the failure of our free market healthcare system to control costs. In contrast to many products and services
we purchase, healthcare simply doesn't lend itself to the comparisons
that transparency allows in a free market. Many factors are involved. The
average person cannot be expected to have knowledge of illness or treatment options to make informed decisions. The dizzying complexity of
both medical care and insurance plan design also precludes the consumer
from making informed choices. Intervening layers within the healthcare
system, consisting of employer plans and plan design, doctors and other
providers, and insurance companies all add complexity that limits and
clouds consumer decisions. And primary care physicians and insurance
company networks strongly influence or dictate choice.

For example, you might select an insurance plan as an individual, or
one offered by your employer, because it has a low price and includes
your doctor in its network. This feels like an informed choice. However,
when you become ill, your doctor, not you, decides if you require surgery,
and your doctor, not you, chooses the hospital you go to. Much to your
surprise the anesthesiologist and radiologist involved in your treatment
are not "in-network" and, as a result, you incur huge bills. Transparency
did not exist beyond choosing your plan and primary doctor. The other
decisions surrounding your treatment were not yours. Studies show that
about two thirds of Americans worry about unexpected healthcare bills.
This is but one example of many in our complex system.

Another example can be drawn from the author's own personal experience. Recently, I was confronted by two health issues. The first involved abdominal pain and bloating and the second related to my heart
functioning.

As abdominal pain and bloating became severe, I called my primary
care physician and my gastroenterologist. They both instructed me to
go to a specific hospital for a CT scan of the abdomen. Then, following
the CT scan, my gastroenterologist sent me for other tests such as an
MRA and MRI at specific testing facilities. From these tests, he then
determined that a blockage in my mesenteric artery was the cause of
my abdominal issues and told me to see a specific vascular surgeon who
would be able to address the issue. That vascular surgeon operated in a
specific hospital only, and it was there that the procedure was performed.
During this episode, the only choice that I made was the selection of

my gastroenterologist. The test providers, the surgeon, and the location of the surgery were all determined starting with my gastroenterologist who I trusted implicitly. I never once thought to question the selections made for me by doctors, and even then, never questioned the choice of surgeons. And because I was covered by fairly comprehensive insurance, I never thought of price issues.

My heart condition followed a similar pattern. My cardiologist ordered a cardiac stress test performed at a specified facility. From the results of the test, he determined that a coronary artery blockage was restricting blood flow to my heart. He instructed me to meet with a specified surgeon who performed the procedure to place a stent in my left descending coronary artery at a hospital that was the only one he accessed to perform operations. The procedure was performed, and I stayed overnight at the same hospital. Here again, as with the abdominal episode, the only choice that I made was the selection of the original doctor, my cardiologist who I trusted completely. The test providers, the surgeon, and the location of the surgery were all determined starting with him. I never once thought to question the selections made for me by doctors, and even then, never questioned the choice of surgeons. And because I was covered by health insurance, I never thought of price issues.

Both of these episodes experienced by the author clearly demonstrate the lack of transparency and patient choice in our current free market healthcare system. This is the major factor in the system's inability to control costs.

The healthcare insurance industry is well aware of the lack of transparency and choice. Wendell Potter, a former executive at CIGNA, one of America's largest healthcare insurers, stated in an Op-Ed he wrote in the *New York Times*, "Americans now have little choice when it comes to managing their healthcare. Most can't choose their own plan or how long they retain it, or even use it to select the doctor or hospital they prefer."[1] He has indicated many times that choice is a public relations concoction. And that lack of a choice is a huge vulnerability in the current system.[2]

In addition to the lack of transparency within our current free market system, the element of human nature, and its relationship to healthcare, is another component that plays a key role in choice.

In the last chapter, we discussed Professor Uwe Reinhardt whose research revealed that it's the prices that drive the high cost of healthcare in the United States. The author has had the great privilege of attending a number Professor Reinhardt's lectures for healthcare and business professionals that he delivered while teaching at Princeton. In one of those lectures, he discussed the element of human nature's role in the choice of doctors and hospitals using his personal experience as a basis.

One pleasant spring morning in Princeton, New Jersey, the Professor was out on the sidewalk in front of his home with his son. He had purchased a bicycle for his son a few months before, fully equipped with training wheels. He had watched his son joyously ride his bike, in the beginning teetering back and forth between the left and right training wheels. After a few weeks or so, his son began to ride steadier, with much less support from the training wheels. Then, soon afterward, it seemed he was riding perfectly upright with no help at all from those noisy training wheels. Observing his son's progress, the professor decided it was time to remove the support and allow his son to ride freely. So, as is the experience of most parents, he removed the training wheels and set out with his son for his first fledgling ride without assistance. Professor Reinhardt, as most parents do, began by holding on to the back of the seat of his son's bike to steady the young rider, providing both physical and emotional support. They moved forward, quite slowly at first, increasing speed with each new ride after resting. When the speed was fast enough, and the Professor judged that his son had achieved the proper balance, he let go of the seat back and watched as his son pedaled confidently with skill and balance, propelling the bike down the street without hesitation.

All went well for a few minutes, but then the unthinkable happened. The boy hit a large bump in the sidewalk and suddenly lost his balance. He began to lose control of his bike, veering to the edge of the path toward the privet hedges and low fences that lined the front yards of homes along the sidewalk. He was still moving along at a brisk pace when his bike grazed the side of a hedge, tossing him out of his seat to the top of the hedge. As he hit the hedge, his momentum caused him to violently role over the top, hitting the ground on the other side with such force that he rolled over and over onto the lawn of a large sprawling Victorian style home. He lay on the ground crying and screaming in pain, blood dripping down his arm from a large gash inflicted when he hit the privet hedge.

From a short distance, Professor Reinhardt observed the calamity and went running down the sidewalk toward his son. Jumping awkwardly over the hedge, the Professor knelt at his now weeping son's side. It was clear from the blood that he had sustained a major wound along his right arm that would no doubt require suturing. More alarming was the condition of his wrist and elbow as his hand hung limply by his side.

The Professor was quite alarmed as he surmised that his son's wrist was probably fractured, and his elbow dislocated. His only thought was to get his son to the closest hospital as quickly as possible to have his arm attended to by a doctor or group of physicians. This was his singular focus. Nothing else mattered. The issue of price or cost never even crossed his mind.

Professor Reinhardt used this rather graphic story to demonstrate that in this set of circumstances, and as he explained, in many less dramatic ones, human nature dictates that concern for loved ones takes precedence over everything else. When one is injured or ill at any level of severity, only securing proper treatment matters. In fact, consideration of cost and price may seem almost profane.

A *New York Times* report in July 2018 entitled "Why Don't We Shop for Health Care?" further explored Professor Reinhardt's research about human nature.[3] Primarily, people don't know what care they need, so they consult a doctor and rely on the doctor's advice on where to go for tests, specialists, and hospitals. This echoes the explanation of the role of primary care physicians in restricting choice of the consumer as explained in the beginning of this chapter.

Furthermore, the report cites a study conducted by the Bureau of National Economic Research which showed that even when given access to a price comparison tool for MRIs, for what the study termed shoppable healthcare like tests, fewer than 1% of patients used it to make a decision. The tool showed that they could save 55% by using the lowest cost provider of the test. The study observed that if people wouldn't shop for an MRI, getting the lowest price, they certainly wouldn't do so with other "shoppable" tests, and certainly would not do so for more complex and variable forms of care. The conclusion: leaving decisions to patients doesn't work.

The study also expands upon the concept presented earlier on this chapter concerning the intervening levels within our current system not being conducive to consumer choice. Here, since most people have insurance that covers MRI testing, they do not view themselves as spending their own money when they need an MRI. Rather, the insurance company is paying, so why care about the price of the test. Even if a copay is attached to the test, it usually is a fixed dollar amount no matter where the test is performed if in the insurance network, unrelated to the price of the test. So, because in most instances, insurance is involved, people don't see that the price of the test is directly affecting them economically. This is human nature at work and as it is compounded by the many layers in our healthcare system.

We can see, as explained in this chapter, there are many factors involved in lack of transparency and choice that are needed to control prices in our current free market healthcare system. As a result, without the price restraints realized through competition, our current free market healthcare system has failed in controlling prices, allowing runaway costs.

Still, aside from healthcare not lending itself to a free market, there are other factors causing higher prices in the United States, including insurance company overhead and administrative costs which we will examine in the next chapter.

Reference List

1 How the Insurance Industry (and I) Invented the 'Choice' Talking Point, by Wendell Potter, *NY Times*, Jan 14, 2020 Opinion. https://www.nytimes.com/2020/01/14/opinion/healthcare-choice-democratic-debate.html?search ResultPosition=7.

2 Deadly Spin: An Insurance Company Insider Speaks Out on How Corporate PR Is Killing Health Care and Deceiving Americans, by Wendell Potter, Bloomsbury Press, Nov 9, 2010.

3 Why We Don't Shop for Healthcare, by Austin Frakt, *New York Times*, Jul 31, 2018, Page B4, https://www.nytimes.com/2018/07/30/upshot/shopping-for-health-care-simply-doesnt-work-so-what-might.html?searchResult Position=1.

4 Overhead and Administrative Costs

To fully understand overhead and administrative costs and gain a perspective of how they affect pricing of healthcare, it is helpful to gain some insight into how insurance companies establish their pricing. The process involved determines how much a consumer or an employer pays for a health plan and is critical in determining deductibles, copays, and insurance networks. The purpose here is not to provide an exhaustive examination, but rather to provide some appreciation for the complexity of insurance pricing and its relationship to overhead and administrative costs within our healthcare system.

Before we begin, it is necessary to review the overall concept of insurance. In essence, this involves spreading risk, in this case healthcare risk, across a group of people, lessening the impact on any individual. Risk is the uncertainty around financial loss. Healthy persons' premiums cover the costs of those individuals needing care. Insurance companies' rates or premiums are driven by the overall health risk of the group being covered, in which the composition of the group cannot be weighted toward higher risk individuals. If so, higher premiums are needed to cover the additional risk and that will cause adverse selection, which happens when insurance premiums increase, and lower risk healthier individuals stop purchasing insurance coverage. The concept of adverse selection is what drove the Individual Mandate of the Affordable Care Act that required healthier younger people to purchase insurance.

After having reviewed overall insurance concepts, next we will explore the components of expected claims. When added to overhead (also called fixed costs or retention), expected claims determine an insurance company's premium rate or what it charges employers or individuals for coverage. An insurance company needs to estimate the claims for the coming year in order to set its prices. To do this, the company uses past paid claims over the prior 12 months as a base point and projects those claims forward into the upcoming year. Paid claims are the total dollars paid to hospitals, doctors, and other healthcare providers. Then, medical cost trend applied to paid claims is used to make the projection for the next year. Trend is the sum of expected medical inflation, demographic changes and health deterioration within the insured group under consideration,

DOI: 10.4324/9781003286271-4

new medical technology and drugs, increased cost for medical services to avoid malpractice, and budgeted spending on advertisement.

The insurer must also calculate incurred but not revealed claims (IBNR). These are claims which have occurred, but because of the time lag resulting from claims recording and processing, have not been accounted for. Insurance companies establish reserves, or money set aside to account for IBNR because if the plan were to terminate, these claims remain as the liability of the insurer. Different insurance companies have their own formulas for estimating IBNR, but since the speed of processing technology has rapidly increased, IBNR has become less important.

Another factor in expected claims is pooling charges for high claims. These are unexpected and unpredictable events. In this category are episodes like premature births that can result in millions of dollars for neonatal intensive care unit charges and the costs of complications that the baby may develop. Pooling charges are mostly included for groups of under 15,000 lives. This is because the smaller the group size, the less reliable projections are, and the more sensitive the overall experience of the group is to a severe health episode that leads to a large increase in claims dollars.

Insurance companies must also consider plan design changes and weigh the effect of fixed dollar copays which increase claims dollars for the company as the cost for any health service increases.

Here, we should mention the concept of loss ratio. This is defined as paid claims divided by premium rate, or the percentage of premium paid by the insurance company for claims. The usual broad target is between 80% for smaller groups with less lives and 90% for larger groups. So, using the loss ratio formula, the amount for retention, or overhead, is typically between 10% and 20% of the insurance company's premium or what it charges for coverage. The Affordable Care Act, passed in 2016, requires an 80% loss ratio. Loss ratio is another element used by insurance companies in establishing rates.

Our purpose above was not to overload the reader with the technical intricacies of insurance company underwriting and processes. In fact, the discussion was a simplified examination, excluding many of the topics associated with establishing rates for employers like retrospective rating, self-funding, self-insurance, risk credibility, and plan rating methodology such as community and group rating, to name a few. Rather, our goal was to help the reader gain some general appreciation for the complexity in determining paid claims and setting prices. All of the work required to develop the rates, as described above, is quite costly and expensive in the form of professional salaries, support staff, office space, and data systems, none of which adds value to patient care. This is important for two main reasons. First is, as we will see in the following discussion of overhead, that complexity drives up insurance companies' operating expenses, the largest component of overhead, that must be recovered in pricing. The main elements of operating expenses propelled upward are salaries, report generation, facilities, and technology. Second is the realization that the complexity, and its cost, is inherent in the operation of every health insurer in the United States. There are many hundreds of insurers in the United States, some have multiple divisions or subsidiaries. As we have seen, the complexity of the processes is a key factor in driving up costs in all of these companies. So, the costs are multiplied many hundreds of times. Additionally, the cost of all the elements of insurance company operation is multiplied many times. So, high cost is driven not just by the complexity of operation individually in each company, but also dramatically compounded by duplication of effort caused by the patchwork of insurance companies. And each insurance company has numerous plans and rate structures which magnify complexity and significantly increase costs even further. These factors are key culprits in the high costs of our free market healthcare system.

Now that we have provided an overview of paid claims, the first factor insurance companies use in establishing premium rates, next we will examine retention, also called fixed costs or overhead, which is the second factor in premium determination, or the price the insurance company charges for coverage.

An insurance company's overhead costs, or retention, consist of operating expenses, commissions, risk charges, premium taxes, and profit. Operating expenses typically include the cost of claims processing, facilities, salaries, customer service, technology, report production, disease management and wellness programs, and network development, and usually represent about 9% of the premium rate when paid claims are 80% of the premium rate (see loss ratio, above). Commissions are typically about 4%. Risk charges, which are a hedge against the possibility that the company's claims estimate is incorrect, is about 3% of premium. State or premium taxes are in the range of 2%, and profit is about 2% or less.[1] Of course, these percentages vary by company.

As discussed above, insurance overhead is a major factor in the cost of high prices of healthcare in the United States. A comparison with insurance overhead costs per capita with other countries in Figure 4.1 highlights this fact.

As Figure 4.1 shows, the health insurance overhead in the United States at $842 per capita is outrageous. It is nearly five times that of Canada at $144 per capita. And over four times that of Holland at $202. While compared with Germany and Switzerland at $273, and France at $279, insurance overhead per capita in the United States is over three times higher.

Next, we will more closely examine the United States compared with Canada for a number of reasons. Canada healthcare is funded through a single-payer system, very much like Medicare For All. Also, Canada and

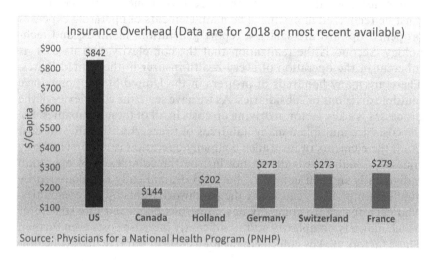

Figure 4.1 Comparing insurance overhead costs to those other countries

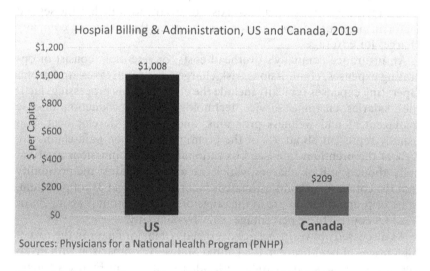

Figure 4.2 A comparison of hospital billing in the United States to those of Canada in 2019

the United States are similar in many other ways in addition to the fact that Canada is a neighboring country, including culture, historical roots, and language.

Figure 4.2 compares hospital billing and administration costs per capita in each country.[2]

The United States, under its free market system, spends nearly five times in hospital billing and administration per capita, $1,008, than Canada spends, $209, under its single-payer healthcare system. These costs are reflected in the higher prices of healthcare in the United States that we explored in Chapter 2.

The huge disparity in these costs is a result of the numerous healthcare insurers, plans, and rate structures in the United States, as we explained previously in this chapter. To illustrate this point, Dr. David Cutler indicated on a PBS news interview, based on data reported in the *Journal of the American Medical Association* (JAMA), in 2018 the Duke Medical Center, one of America's premier hospitals employed 1,600 billing clerks for just under 1,000 beds, more than one billing clerk per hospitalized patient![3] An icon in American Healthcare, the Cleveland Clinic, reported the following in Modern Healthcare of September 30, 2019:

> Compounding the complexity, we have many different payers and multiple different products within each payer. Specifically, we estimate that we have 3,000 contracted rate schedules across the Cleveland Clinic ... system. Further, our chargemaster reflects over 70,000 lines .... Thus, the number of data points needed to be posted would exceed 210 million ....[4]

The Duke Medical Center's and The Cleveland Clinic's information are indicative of the waste and duplication in America's current free market healthcare system. Since the information is focused on hospital settings, it is also important to examine the effect of our free market system on doctor's administrative costs.

Figure 4.3 compares physicians' billing-related expenses per capita in the United States with those in Canada.[2]

Physicians' billing-related expenses in the United States are over five times higher than in Canada. This again, as in hospitals, is the result of the number of insurance companies, plans, and rate structures in the United States.

If we compare overall administrative costs per capita, the same picture emerges caused by the same set of factors, which by now should be of no surprise to the reader. Figure 4.4 indicates that overall healthcare administrative costs per capita in the United States are just over four times the cost in Canada per capita.[2]

As Drs. Steffie Woolhandler and David Himmelstein point out in the May 31, 2019 edition of the JAMA, "The current, fragmented payment system entails complexity that adds no value. Physicians and hospitals must navigate contracting and credentialing with multiple plans and contend with numerous payment rates and restrictions, preauthorization requirements, quality metrics, and formularies."[5]

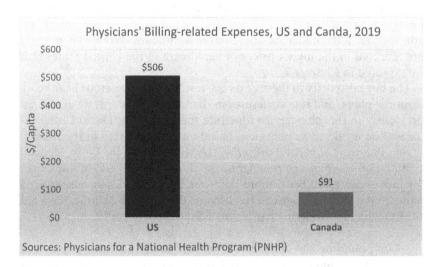

Figure 4.3 Comparing physicians' billing-related expenses United States versus those in Canada, 2019

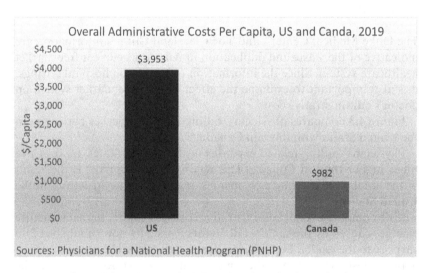

Figure 4.4 Overall healthcare administrative costs in the United States versus Canada, 2019

Jeffrey Sachs, world-renowned professor of economics, senior UN advisor, and University Professor, the highest academic rank at Columbia University, stated in his review of a University of Massachusetts Study of Medicare For All, "Medicare For All promises a system that is fairer, more efficient, and vastly less expensive than America's bloated, monopolized, over-priced and under-performing private health insurance system. America spends far more on health care and gets far less for its money than any other high-income country...Medicare For All offers a proven and wholly workable way forward."[6]

Reference List

1 Underwriting for Medical Plans, course presented by the Philadelphia Employee Benefits Association at Independence Blue Cross, Maureen Lee and Elizabeth Patterson speakers.
2 Costs of health care administration in the United States and Canada. Steffie Woolhandler, Terry Campbell, and David U Himmelstein, *NE Journal of Medicine*, Aug 23, 2003, https://pubmed.ncbi.nlm.nih.gov/12930930/.
3 Why Does Health Care Cost So Much in America? Ask Harvard's David Cutler, by David Cutler, *PBS Newshour Economy*, Nov 19, 2013, 5:23 EDT, https://www.pbs.org/newshour/economy/why-does-health-care-cost-so-m.
4 Modern Healthcare, September 30, 2019, as reported by Physicians for a National Health Plan, Short Slide Deck 2019.
5 Single-Payer Reform – Medicare For All, by Stephie Woolhandler and David U. Himmelstein, Viewpoint Health Policy, Published Online, May 31, 2019, and reproduced on the PNHP website.
6 Reviewer Assessments of Economic analysis of Medicare For All, Political Economy Research Institute of the University of Massachusetts Amherst, September 2017 review, https://peri.umass.edu/reviewer-assessments-of-economic-analysis-of-medicare-for-all.

5   The Burden of High Healthcare Costs

In the prior chapters, we have defined the magnitude of the extremely high healthcare costs in America and have examined the underlying causes and reasons for those costs. In this chapter, we will explore the economic burden such costs place on the population as the result of expanding medical debt. We will also consider the pressures these costs place on employers that provide healthcare coverage for between 160 million and 170 million residents of this country.

As indicated in Chapter 2, it's important to understand that no one is immune from escalating healthcare costs. Even for those who are fortunate to be covered by employer plans, a 2020 Kaiser Family Foundation Survey reported that the amount an employee pays for her/his healthcare coverage averages $5,600 a year for family coverage with an average deductible of $1,650 annually.[1] In fact, a 2020 US Bureau of Labor Statistics survey of employee healthcare costs shows that family coverage for those covered by employer plans was $6,800 annually.[2] This amount is over $1,000 higher than the Kaiser survey probably because of the survey's participant mix, leaning more heavily toward smaller employers which pay more for coverage. These costs have been raising every year and continue to escalate, representing a significant economic burden for many Americans. Since 2010, these premiums have risen by about 50%, more than double the rise in wages or inflation, and are even affecting many former "Cadillac plans" under which employee contributions have been historically low or nonexistent.

Some 30 million Americans are uninsured and without health insurance coverage protection against medical costs.[3] And many of those with insurance are dangerously exposed to the high costs of medical care resulting from a number of factors. First, as mentioned above, is the escalating costs of insurance premiums and high deductibles even in the best of coverage plans. Then, because of the high cost of quality coverage, many are driven to less expensive high deductible plans, where the economic exposure is quite substantial before the deductible is met. There is also the issue of many plans that cover only a certain percentage of the cost of care. Even in high-quality plans, 80/20 cost-sharing in which

DOI: 10.4324/9781003286271-5

a person is responsible for 20% of the costs is not unusual. With ever increasing healthcare costs, that 20% amount in actual dollars continues to grow each year. Also, there is the issue of surprise billing as explained in Chapter 2, where for reasons beyond a person's control they are billed by a medical provider or facility outside of the network of their insurance company. Although the Biden Administration is addressing this issue, it still remains problematic. Lastly, recently exacerbated by the COVID-19 pandemic, is the folly of tying healthcare coverage to employment. As people leave a job because of downsizing and layoffs among other reasons, they are exposed to the potential of catastrophic medical costs in between jobs. COBRA, the Consolidated Omnibus Budget Reconciliation Act, gives employees who lose their health benefits the right to continue coverage for a limited period of time, but is frequently too expensive because the employee typically is required to pay the full amount of the insurance without their employer's contribution. And the benefit can expire before the employee obtains another job.

So, for all of the reasons outlined above, Americans bear the weight of the high cost of healthcare in the United States which has become a major contributing factor in many bankruptcies.

The Commonwealth Fund reported that many adults in the United States are faced with medical debt problems: 43% had used up all their savings to pay their bills, 43% had received a lower credit rating as a result of their debt, 32% strained credit card debt, and 18% said they had delayed education or career plans.[4]

A recent survey entitled "The Burden of Medical Debt: Results from the Kaiser Family Foundation/New York Times Medical Bills Survey" by L. Hamel et al. presented revealing information about the issue of the economic burden of high healthcare costs.[5] It reported that nearly one quarter of Americans within the age group of 18–64 experience problems paying medical bills. Among those with medical bill problems, nearly half indicate that the bills have had a major impact on their families. And although those with lower incomes are more likely than higher income people to report problems paying medical bills, among those who had problems paying medical bills, those with higher incomes are just as likely to report that the bills had a major impact. And the survey shows that while insurance may initially protect people from having medical bills problems, once the problems develop, the consequences are quite similar regardless of insurance status. This is displayed in Figure 5.1.

The survey also reported the sacrifices that households made in a year as a result of the debt they had incurred because of healthcare costs. The percentages are shown below in Table 5.1, including reducing spending on food and clothing, taking an extra job, depleting savings, borrowing money, withdrawing money from retirement and savings accounts, taking out a second mortgage, and seeking aid from a charity.

Over Four in Ten with Medical Bill Problems Report a Major Impact on Their Family

AMONG THOSE WHO HAD PROBLEMS PAYING HOUSEHOLD MEDICAL BILLS IN THE PAST 12 MONTHS: Overall, how much of an impact have these medical bills had on you and your family?

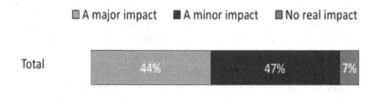

By Insurance Status

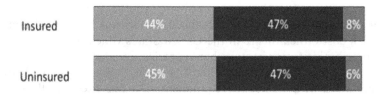

NOTE: Don't know/Refused responses not shown.
SOURCE: Kaiser Family Foundation/New York Times Medical Bills Survey (conducted August 28-September 28, 2015)

Figure 5.1 Kaiser Family Foundation survey results (2015) showing that four in ten people are severely impacted by medical bills

Table 5.1 Percent of survey respondents indicating have done each of the following activities in order to pay medical bills

Put off vacations or other major household purchases	72%
Cut back spending on food, clothing, or basic household items	70%
Used up all or most of savings	59%
Taken an extra job or worked more hours	41%
Borrowed money from friends or family	37%
Increased credit card debt	34%
Taken money out of retirement, college, or other long-term savings accounts	26%
Changed your living situation	17%
Taken out another type of loan	15%
Borrowed money from a payday lender	13%
Sought the aid of a charity or non-profit organization	12%
Taken out another mortgage on home	2%
Made other significant changes to way of life	15%

To complement this chart and illustrate in real-life terms the sacrifices people make in order to pay medical bills, the survey reported the meaningful changes made in their lives using the participants own words. These sacrifices, in survey participants' words, are summarized by the following:

- "Apartment instead of house. Not getting groceries some weeks to get by."
- "Charges for my insulin exceeded $1,200 a month (three times the amount of my house payment). I had to reduce the amount of insulin I took based on what I could afford; my health was negatively impacted as a result."
- "Cold showers, can't fix plumbing. Other needed repairs have been patched as best as possible but not fixed."
- "Medical Insurance/bills was the deciding factor in a job change. I gave up other benefits to choose a job that had the best medical coverage."
- "Sold everything we could spare."
- "Can't take the kids anywhere. Wish I could do more for my kids!"
- "I need physical therapy after shoulder repair, but I couldn't afford to finish it. I wish I could have."
- "I am losing my house."
- "I've cut back on just about everything for my family and the way we live."

Many of the very brief statements are quite troublesome and distressing, revealing the severe impact that healthcare costs have on American families.

The survey also reported the share of total debt that healthcare bills represent, shown in Figure 5.2. Using the chart, we can calculate that about half of those with medical debt indicate that the debt represents about 50% or more of their total debt, aside from mortgage payments.

Additionally, healthcare bills can also lead to problems in paying for basic necessities and/or meeting different financial obligations. As shown in Figure 5.3, about 60% of those with medical bill problems indicated they experienced difficulty paying other bills because of medical debt. Even more seriously, about a third indicated they were unable to pay for basic necessities. The survey also reports that about 25% of those with medical bills were contacted by a collection agency.

Additionally, in April 2021, a report authored by Neil Bennett et al. about the burden of medical debt published by the US Census Bureau revealed that about 20% of US households could not afford to pay for

Share of Total Debt Due to Medical Bills

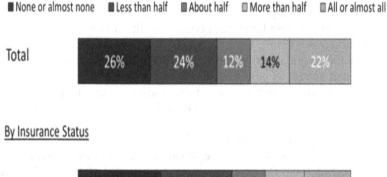

AMONG THOSE WHO HAD PROBLEMS PAYING HOUSEHOLD MEDICAL BILLS IN THE PAST 12 MONTHS: Not counting your mortgage, what share of your total debt would you estimate is due to medical bills?

■ None or almost none   ■ Less than half   ■ About half   ▢ More than half   ▢ All or almost all

Total

| 26% | 24% | 12% | 14% | 22% |

By Insurance Status

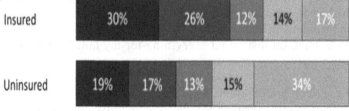

Insured

| 30% | 26% | 12% | 14% | 17% |

Uninsured

| 19% | 17% | 13% | 15% | 34% |

NOTE: All or almost all includes those who still owe money for medical bills and have no other loans or debts. None or almost none includes those who have paid off all medical bills. Don't know/Refused responses not shown. SOURCE: Kaiser Family Foundation/New York Times Medical Bills Survey (conducted August 28-September 28, 2015)

Figure 5.2 Kaiser Family Foundation survey results (2015) showing total debt represented by healthcare bills

medical care up front or when they received care. Among households with medical debt, the median amount owed was $2,000.[6]

Households with children under age 18 (24.7%) were more likely than those without children (16.5%) to carry medical debt, and over 12% were unable to pay their mortgage or rent.

Lastly, in November 2019, CNBC reported that about 140 million Americans had faced financial hardship because of medical costs that year. It also reported that high healthcare bills were the No. 1 reason people considered taking money out of their retirement accounts or filing for bankruptcy.[7]

Reports of Difficulty Paying Other Bills and Basic Needs As A Result Of Medical Bills

AMONG THOSE WHO HAD PROBLEMS PAYING HOUSEHOLD MEDICAL BILLS IN THE PAST 12 MONTHS: Percent who say they have experienced any of the following in the past 12 months as a result of these medical bills:

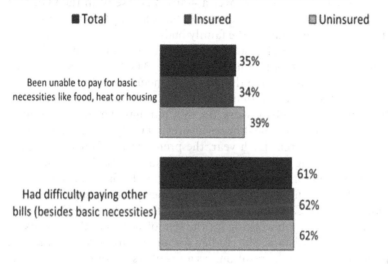

SOURCE: Kaiser Family Foundation/New York Times Medical Bills Survey (conducted August 28-September 28, 2015)

Figure 5.3 Kaiser Family Foundation survey results (2015) showing that as a result of medical bills, reports of difficulty paying other bills and basic needs

    In order to better understand the data and numbers reviewed in this chapter thus far, and bring them to life, it is helpful to review the stories of a few families who have experienced the high cost of healthcare and medical debt. We will begin with the less severe, but still impactful, issues of increasing premium cost and then progress to stories of those who experienced illnesses that resulted in extreme economic hardship.

    First are two stories related to the author through recent interviews. Both families preferred to remain anonymous for various reasons and I certainly respect their wishes by referring to them as Mr. Jones and Ms. Smith.[8]

    Mr. Jones is a scientist employed by a state government agency. He made the decision a number of years ago to work for the state because of the outstanding benefits package it provided its employees, including a fully paid "Cadillac" medical plan with a limited deductible and minimal or no copays. He was well aware of the fact that his salary was lower than he could have earned at other private organizations, but the attraction of the strong benefits package offered by the state was paramount in his choice of employer. Unfortunately, for Mr. Jones and his family, his state employer has reacted to the rising cost of healthcare by passing costs on to their employees. Mr. Jones now pays more than $8,000 a year for his medical benefits, and with increasing deductibles and copays, that amount is even higher. This is over a 400% increase from the plan that attracted him to work for the state only ten years ago and represents a real and continuing strain on the family budget.

Ms. Smith also related her story of economic pressure from healthcare costs, this time resulting in a lifestyle change. Ms. Smith is a hairstylist working in a hair salon, a job that typically includes health insurance as a benefit. Her husband, a self-employed contractor, also had no access to health insurance through his work. So, they purchased medical insurance privately through a major healthcare insurer, a family plan covering them and their three children. Each year, the premium for their private plan kept increasing along with their deductibles and copays. Finally, when the monthly family premium reached nearly $1,500, the Smiths could not afford to continue their coverage. Since they knew with three children that they could not just continue on with no healthcare coverage, Ms. Smith was forced to take a job working for the school system in their township as an Education Assistant. She studied for months to pass the exam that was a requirement for the position. As a result, as a mother of three, she works two jobs, as an Educational Assistant from 8 am to 4 pm and then drives to her second job as a hairstylist working many nights until nine or ten o'clock and on Saturdays. Her children miss her, but that's the price she and her family must pay in lifestyle to afford healthcare insurance.

Another story is that of Bliss Butler, reported in a research interview with CNBC.[7] She is 59, lives outside of Oklahoma City and is employed at an area museum. Ms. Butler lost her job in 2013, and as a result, she became uninsured because it was difficult to make her COBRA medical continuation payments. Then, she experienced several health crises. First, Ms. Butler developed a kidney stone, necessitating a trip to the emergency room followed by a hospital stay. Then, a follow-up visit to a surgery center was required to remove a stent.

To add insult to injury, she then broke her leg. Because she was still in debt from her previous medical bills, she avoided taking an ambulance to a hospital. Ms. Butler had to have surgery to repair her broken leg which cost the large sum of $60,000 for which she was billed. And if this wasn't enough, she had a huge scare when she experienced heart palpitations, which required yet another emergency room visit.

After all of this, Ms. Butler openly admits that she doesn't know the entire amount of her medical debt. Separate invoices of large amounts have appeared with striking dollar amounts, like $36,860.75 and $19,881.58. She has explained that it is quite difficult to understand what specifically these amounts are billing her for, as well as the actual dollar amount she really owes. She has already spent all of the $20,000 she had accumulated in her retirement savings. Ms. Butler has never been on any kind of public assistance, including Medicaid, and is very proud of the fact that she has always worked for a living.

Quite unfortunately, Ms. Butler's next step is likely filing for bankruptcy. And that's after years of working, avoiding accumulating debts, and being careful with her money.

"I don't think that my particular story is that unusual," she said. "There are so many people that are in the same position that I am."

In reaction to Bliss Butlers story and others, Dr. Marty Makary, Professor at Johns Hopkins University Medical School remarked, "The great public trust in America's health care institutions is being eroded. The price gauging and predatory billing today is threatening the great public trust in the medical profession. We have an irrational marketplace..."[9]

Then, there is the story of Debbie Moehnke as reported in Time Magazine of March 2019, entitled "She owed $227,000 in Medical Bills - Even With Insurance. Here's What it Took to Pay Them."[10] Ms. Moehnke was struck by a massive heart attack while she waited in a Vancouver, Washington medical clinic in 2018.

Larry Moehnke, her husband explained, "She had an appointment because her feet were swollen real bad. But she got in there and it was like, 'I can't breathe, I can't breathe!'"

Ms. Moehnke, 59 years old, was rushed by ambulance to a local hospital, where she was stabilized. The next day she was transferred to Oregon Health & Science University in Portland to get urgent cardiac care.

The treatment consisted of heart bypass surgery, the replacement of one heart valve and the repair of second valve. Unfortunately, after her recovery from the procedures, Ms. Moehnke developed a severe infection requiring antibiotics delivered intravenously. That treatment necessitated a month's stay in the hospital, some of it in intensive care. After curing the infection, she was discharged and sent home.

Much to the Moehnke's surprise, they received bills exceeding $450,000 for Ms. Moehnke's surgery, treatment, and hospital stay. After her health insurance paid its share of the bill, they were informed that they owed over $225,000 of the total amount.

After learning about the amount owed, Ms. Moehnke lamented, "I wish I would have known. I would have said 'no' to life support. We'll lose everything."

MSNBC.com reported stories about families facing economic issues because of medical bills, and that even good health insurance is no guarantee of coverage or protection against high bills for care. One particular story is best told as directly reported by MSNBC.[11]

"Before their second child was born, Courtney and Isaac Elliott shunned most things medical and didn't understand why anyone wouldn't. They had a healthy little girl, Aniyah, now five, and good insurance provided by Aetna through Isaac's job."

"I ate all organic and I never took any medicine and I had a medication-free birth," said Courtney Elliott, who goes by the nickname "Courey." "I had my baby at home."

Linden arrived on Dec. 15, 2006, a dark-haired, dark-eyed baby who within days revealed severe problems. He had trouble breathing and needed surgery to correct a malformed larynx.

He couldn't swallow well, and breast milk wound up in his lungs instead of his stomach. Within weeks, he needed to be fed solely through a tube. Other puzzling problems emerged as well: he couldn't regulate his body temperature, he had trouble with motor skills, his bowels didn't work right.

Results of a muscle biopsy confirmed his parents' worst fears: Linden had mitochondrial disease, a rare genetic disorder that often leads to severe disability – and death.

"He could live 10 years or he could live 10 days," Elliott said of Linden's prognosis.

The disease results from the failure of the mitochondria, the part of human cells responsible for processing oxygen and energy.

It's a devastating medical diagnosis that conjures for parents an endless cycle of care. And it's a devastating financial diagnosis as well.

"It's not possible, emotionally or financially, to prepare to have a child as ill as Linden," said Linden's specialist, Dr. Mary Kay Koenig.

The family must travel from Tennessee to Texas at their own expense three or four times a year to see Koenig, one of the nation's few specialists in mitochondrial disease.

At first, the family thought the medical expenses would be no problem. Isaac Elliott earns $72,000 a year at Bechtel Jacobs and his generous insurance covers 100% of services after initial co-payments.

But like many families coping with chronic illness, the Elliotts were surprised to learn that the copays for Linden's condition would be extensive, unrelenting – and a constant financial drain.

"Each time he has a tube change, it's $150. Each hospital visit is $250. Each emergency room visit is $100. Each surgical procedure is $100," Elliott said. "In the past 30 days, we've had two ER visits, a hospital stay, his prescriptions."

The Elliotts spend at least $2,000 a month on out-of-pocket costs for Linden's care, and often more. That leaves little for anything but the most basic family expenses – and sometimes not even those.

"I didn't pay my electric bill this month and I didn't pay my gas bill this month," admits Elliott, who must stay home to take care of Linden. "We live paycheck to paycheck."

They've managed to buy a tidy house in a vine-covered east Tennessee neighborhood, thanks to a no-down-payment loan, but their furniture is well-worn and sparse. They rarely eat out, except when they're in the hospital, and they confine family outings to free trips to playgrounds or parks.

There are times, Elliott adds, when she can't afford all of Linden's medications, even with generous help from relatives.

"There's no worse feeling than having to weigh your child's needs vs. what you can afford," she said.

Still, Linden is hardly the sum of his symptoms. The sturdy, 34-pound toddler has a quick smile and verbal skills that test at a four-year-old's level. His vocabulary includes words like "duodenum," and he proudly shows off his stuffed ape, Chunky Monkey, who also sports a hospital bracelet and a tube in his tummy.

When he gets a little wild, Linden will hitch a ride on his IV stand, scooting with one foot, then rolling down a hospital hallway.

When the deep dimples fade, however, there are often flashes of pain. Linden tires quickly, retreating to the comfort of a pacifier and his mother's arms.

"Owie!" the toddler cries as a nurse tests his blood to prepare for surgery. "I don't like pokes!"

An operation on Oct. 12 was aimed at installing a port in Linden's shoulder to allow fast regulation of his blood sugar. Without it, his glucose level has been vacillating wildly, creating constant risk of coma – or death.

Elliott says she never knows whether to expect a normal day or an emergency. Some children with mitochondrial disease have lived to adulthood, but others die very young.

"I think it's very difficult for me as a mom to know that there's nothing I can do," she said. "I can try my best and he still might die. That is just an incredibly powerless feeling."

On top of all that worry is the crushing financial burden.

"That's the kicker," she said. "You got the crappy end of the lottery and you got a medically fragile child and you'll have to fight for his life. And now, we're going to drain you financially, too."

Health reform could ease the Elliott's financial worries, if not the medical concerns, said Nichols, the health economist. The proposals under consideration mandating that virtually everyone purchase health insurance could boost the pool of potential payers and allow new limits on out-of-pocket costs.

For the Elliotts, such limits could be far lower than the $25,000 or more a year they now pay.

"You could afford that because you could get everybody in the pool," Nichols said. "To make the pool reflect the whole population, it'll be, on average, cheaper."

Any change would be welcome, said Elliott, who supports a government-funded public health insurance option.

"If my husband were to lose his job, we'd be broke in a week," she said, adding later: "So few people understand they could be next."

Perhaps, the most famous story of all was broadcast on ABC's late-night talk show, "Jimmy Kimmel Live" on May 1, 2017, during his opening monologue.[12]

Telling the story of his son who shortly after birth needed surgery for congenital heart defects and within the debates about coverage under the Affordable Care Act (ACA) Mr. Kimmel wept and while looking directly into the television camera spoke in a broken voice.

He described the recent birth of his son. Struggling with his words, he told the story. Within hours of his son's birth, a nurse noticed that he was purple and whisked him away for observation.

"Now more doctors and nurses and equipment come in, and it's a terrifying thing," he said. "My wife is back in the recovery room, she has no idea what's going on, and I'm standing in a room full of worried-looking people." The medical team's diagnosis was that his son, Billy, had a congenital heart defect, so he was rushed into emergency surgery.

"It was the longest three hours of my life," he said, weeping. Fortunately, the procedure was successful, and Billy recovered, though he'll need more surgeries. Mr. Kimmel then went on to thank the nurses and doctors on his son's case. Most importantly, he acknowledged that while his son will likely be just fine, many families are still at Children's Hospital Los Angeles and suffering, many depending on funds that President Trump proposed be cut from the federal budget. He said, "more than 40% of the people who would have been affected by those cuts to the National Institute of Health are children."

Mr. Kimmel, continued,

> We were brought up to believe that we live in the greatest country in the world, but until a few years ago (apparently referring to times before the passage of the Affordable Care Act) millions and millions of us had no access to health insurance at all. Before 2014, if you were born with congenital heart disease like my son was, there was a good chance you would never be able to get health insurance because you had a pre-existing condition. You were born with a pre-existing condition, and if your parents didn't have medical insurance, you might not even live long enough to get denied because of a pre-existing condition.
>
> "If your baby is going to die, and it doesn't have to, it shouldn't matter how much money you make," Kimmel said, insisting that the issue shouldn't be divisive. "Let's stop with the nonsense. This isn't football; there are no teams. We are the team; it's the United States. Don't let their partisan squabbles divide us on something every decent person wants. We need to care for each other."

Most poignantly, he concluded: "No parent should ever have to decide if they can afford to save their child's life. It just shouldn't happen. Not here."

The above stories are just a few of the multitudes that illustrate, in real-life terms, the problems of our broken free market healthcare system and the very high costs associated with it, placing tremendous burdens on average Americans.

Next, we will overview the burden of runaway healthcare costs on employers who provide medical plans for their employees. Certainly not in the same category of the personal stories just related, yet they provide another perspective of the impact of high and runaway healthcare costs.

The annual Kaiser Family Foundation Survey 2020 reported that for the year 2020, the total cost of a health plan covering a family was $21,342, with employees paying $5,588, or about a quarter of that amount.[1] This resulted in employers paying nearly $16,000 annually per employee for family coverage. Such a huge burden has been increasing dramatically for years and has grown by over 50% in the past ten years. Between 160 and 170 million Americans were covered by these plans before the pandemic during which millions lost their jobs.

To illustrate in real terms the impact of these numbers, we will relate the author's experience in designing and managing healthcare plans for major corporations as part of the annual "dance" typically occurring as the C-Suite develops the company's budget for the following year. The responsibility falls on the Director of Benefits and the Chief Human Resources Officer (CHO) to propose the budget for providing employee healthcare plans. Part of this process is to project total healthcare costs and then determine how much of this ever-increasing expense will be passed on to employees in the form of premiums deducted from their paycheck to the deductibles and copays they will pay when using the plans for care.

Each year before the budget meetings, light tension builds between the CHO and the Chief Financial Officer (CFO). The CHO is charged with the overall responsibility of attracting, motivating, and retaining employees. Inherently, this charter would dictate that the lower the costs passed on to employees for the company's provided healthcare benefit, the better. In contrast, the CFO is focused on controlling company costs to help sustain and increase the profitability of the company, and therefore, her/his interest is sharing healthcare costs with employees to the greatest extend that is reasonable/possible. The somewhat competing goals of the CHO and the CFO make for lively and frequently strained discussions between them at the C-Suite budget meetings. Depending on the decision style of the organization and after hearing the arguments on both sides, the decision is made either directly by the Chief Executive Officer (CEO) or by an agreement to the appropriate amounts by the members of the C-Suite. Many times, the Director of Benefits proposes additional ways to reduce healthcare costs through creative negotiation processes with insurers or other financial approaches under self-insured plans as well as vehicles like wellness programs. These become part of the discussion at the C-Suite budget meetings.

Most of this activity requires the time, attention, and effort within the CHO's staff, the CFO's staff, and others within the company. And little, if any, of these resources adds to the company's sales or profits which directly affect shareholders and employees, all caused by high and escalating healthcare costs.

Smaller companies bear an equal if not greater burden than larger corporations because they do not have the negotiating leverage with insurance companies that larger corporations have as a result of their size, which also keeps self-insurance and other more cost-effective approaches out of their reach. Also, they have fewer assets to absorb the impact of increasing costs.

A case in point is Richard Master, founder and owner of MCSI, a leader in the picture frame and decorative mirror business. He has been impacted by escalating healthcare costs to such a degree that he produced a video entitled "Fix It" which can be viewed online, as well as brochures and pamphlets that outline the issues of our current free market system and demonstrate the cost-effectiveness of a one-payer system like Medicare For All. Mr. Master has become a leading business advocate and activist for Medicare For All.[13]

His video shows that the costs to provide healthcare as a benefit to his employees had doubled over a number of years, more than any other expense of his business. And despite the cost, the plan his company was able to purchase left employees exposed economically because of the premium cost-sharing and deductibles and copays associated with the plan. The video tells the story of an employee whose spouse becomes critically ill, resulting in healthcare costs that are a terrible economic burden, placing them in severe financial trouble. And this even in the face of the healthcare coverage Mr. Master's company provided. He expresses his concern for his employees, finding their situation and that of his company unacceptable.

Another interesting and telling story about business and healthcare, illustrating both escalating healthcare costs and the complexity of our free market system, is the venture that three giants of industry formed to address the high costs of healthcare. Haven, the venture's name, was formed by CEOs Warren Buffet of Berkshire Hathaway, Jamie Dimon of JP Morgan Chase, and Jeff Bezos of Amazon. The companies, experiencing the high and escalating costs of healthcare, announced the venture in January 2018 to develop ways to lower costs for the three companies while providing high-quality healthcare for their employees. The announcement of the venture was so powerful given the three companies participating, shares of healthcare companies dropped in anticipation of how the combined strength of industry leaders in finance and technology would change the system and reduce costs. Then, only one year later, the venture was ended.

According to the Harvard Business Review, Haven was unable to force the market disruption it hoped to achieve, blocked by profitable insurers and providers.[14] In considering why the entity failed, experts and observers believe the task of forcing market disruption of the complex, many layered, and highly profitable American healthcare system was too daunting. The failure could well be a marker of how difficult it is to attack the convoluted, entrenched, and inefficient system of free market American healthcare. Additionally, the variations and complexity of each company's numerous plans created roadblocks to progress.

Next, we will explore two examples of the burden of high healthcare costs beyond money that consider the ultimate burden – death. First is a study by the federal government reporting that from 2019 to 2020 during the coronavirus pandemic, African American and Hispanic Americans suffered a far steeper drop in life expectancy than white Americans. As reported in the *New York Times* of July 22, 2021, Hispanic and Black Americans experienced a decline in life expectancy of about three years, while whites experienced a decline of only 1.2 years.[15] A number of factors were involved in the disparity, but "deep racial and ethnic inequities in access to health" was one key factor described by Dr. Mary Bassett, professor of health at Harvard University. The *Times* emphasized "the differences in overall health and available care" as a key factor.

Perhaps, even more striking is a 2009 study by a research team at Harvard Medical School which estimated that 2,266 US military veterans under the age of 65 died in 2008 because they lacked health insurance and as a result access to healthcare.[16] They found that 1,461,615 veterans between the ages of 18 and 64 were uninsured in 2008. Veterans were classified as uninsured if they neither had health insurance nor received ongoing care at Veterans Health Administration (VA) hospitals or clinics.

In commenting about the study, Dr. S. Woolhandler, a professor at Harvard Medical School, explained, "Like other uninsured Americans, most uninsured vets are working people – too poor to afford private coverage but not poor enough to qualify for Medicaid or means-tested VA care." She explained further that while many Americans believe all veterans can get care from the VA, even combat veterans may not be able to obtain Veterans Administration care.

Dr. D. Himmelstein, the co-author of the analysis and associate professor of medicine at Harvard, commented, "We should honor.... the more than 2,200 veterans who were killed by our broken health insurance system." This is the ultimate failure of our free market for profit healthcare system, a burden borne by those who served our country and sacrificed so much for all Americans.

Reference List

1 Kaiser Family Foundation 2020 Employer Health Benefits Survey, Published: Oct 08, 2020 https://www.kff.org/health-costs/report/2020-employer-health-benefits-survey/.

2 US Bureau of Labor Statistics US. Department of Labor, The Economics Daily, from Annual Employee Benefits Survey, https://www.bls.gov/opub/ted/2020/average-employee-medical-premium-6797-dollars-for-family-coverage-in-2020.htm.

3 National Health Interview Survey, Health Insurance Coverage, Center for disease Control and Prevention, National Center of Health Statistics, https://www.cdc.gov/nchs/fastats/health-insurance.htm.

4 Testimony: The Growing Cost Burden of Employer Health Insurance for U.S. Families and Implications for Their Health and Economic Security, Testimony, The Commonwealth Fund before the U.S. House of Representatives Committee on Ways and Means, Subcommittee on Select Revenue Measures, Hearing on "How Middle-Class Families Are Faring in Today's Economy," Feb 13, 2019, https://www.commonwealthfund.org/publications/2019/feb/testimony-growing-cost-burden-employer-health-insurance.

5 The Burden of Medical Debt: Results from the Kaiser Family Foundation/New York Times Medical Bills Survey, Liz Hamel, Mira Norton, Karen Pollitz, Larry Levitt, Gary Claxton, and Mollyann Brodie, Jan 5, 2016, https://www.kff.org/health-costs/report/the-burden-of-medical-debt-results-from-the-kaiser-family-foundationnew-york-times-medical-bills-survey/view/print/.

6 19% of U.S. Households Could Not Afford to Pay for Medical Care Right Away, US Census Bureau, Neil Bennett, Jonathan Eggelston, Laryssa Mykyta, and Briana Sullivan, Apr 7, 2021, https://www.census.gov/library/stories/2021/04/who-had-medical-debt-in-united-states.html.

7 137 Million Americans Are Struggling with Medical Debt. Here's What to Know If You Need Some Relief, by Lorie Konish, CNBC Published, Nov 10, 2019 at 9:45 AM, Updated Nov 12, 2019 at 10:53 AM.

8 Interviews with Ken Lefkowitz on Feb 10, 2020. Interviewees Requested Anonymity.

9 Hospital Price Gouging Shows It's Time for Physicians to "Take Back Their Profession," Catalyst Health Network, Oct 24, 2019, https://www.catalysthealthnetwork.com/project-healthcare/2020/8/10/hospital-price-gouging-shows-its-time-for-physicians-to-take-back-their-profession.

10 She Owed $227,000 in Medical Bills-Even with Insurance. Here's What It Took to Pay Them, *Time Magazine*, by Jones Aleccia/*Kaiser Health News*, Mar 21, 2019, https://time.com/5555988/medical-bills-out-of-network/.

11 No Guarantees: 3 Tales of Insurance Disaster, by Jonel Aleccia, Oct 26, 2009 6:24 Am, *MSNBC News*, https://www.nbcnews.com/id/wbna33441437.

12 Jimmy Kimmel Live, ABC, May 1, 2017, https://www.youtube.com/watch?v=MmWWoMcGmo0.

13 Fix It, Healthcare at the Tipping Point, a Movie by Richard Master, https://fixithealthcare.com/watch-the-movie/ and presentation and brochures distributed by Richard Master at an SJNOW and NJ Universal Healthcare Coalition hosted meeting in Mar 30, 2016.

14 Health Care Venture Comes to a Quiet End, by Emily Flitter and Karen Weise, *NY Times*, Jan 5, 2021, https://www.nytimes.com/2021/01/04/business/haven-amazon-berkshire-hathaway-jpmorgan.html?searchResultPosition=1.

15 Virus Widens a Racial Gap in Longevity, by Julie Boseman, Sophie Kasakove, and Daniel Victor, *NY Times*, Jul 22, 2021, https://www.nytimes.com/2021/07/21/us/american-life-expectancy-report.html?search ResultPosition=1.
16 Lack of Health Care Killed 2,266 US Veterans Last Year, *PNHP Newsletter*, Nov 11, 2009, http://www.pnhp.org/news/2009/november/lack_of_health_care_.php.

6 Savings under Medicare For All

In the prior chapters, we examined the duplicative and wasteful costs of insurance company operations as well as the industry's effect on the administrative and billing costs of doctors and hospitals. None of these costs add value to patient care or the overall quality of healthcare in the United States. We have also reviewed the economic burden of high healthcare costs inherent in our current system as it affects families and employers who provide healthcare coverage.

In this chapter, we will explore the cost savings that can be realized from moving away from America's current free market system to Medicare For All, a single-payer system similar to Canada's National Health Plan, NHP.

We begin with the graph in Figure 6.1 comparing healthcare costs as a percent of gross domestic product (GDP).[1] The graph compares the

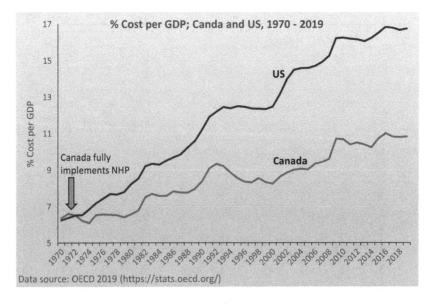

Figure 6.1 Health costs as a percentage of GDP: United States and Canada, 1970–2019

DOI: 10.4324/9781003286271-6

healthcare costs of single-payer system with a free market system, both before its implementation and then afterward over many years.

GDP is all the money spent on goods and services in a given period, used as a general measure of a country's economy. Using costs as a percent of GDP levels the playing field in terms of the size of a country's economy. The period covered is 1970 to 2019 comparing Canada and the United States. The graph is very revealing. It presents a comparison of the cost of the free market system in the United States to a single-payer system in Canada. The Canadian National Health System (NHP on the graph) is referred to as Medicare by many Canadians.

A few very notable observations begin in 1970 prior to Canada adopting its single-payer system. The reader can clearly see that healthcare costs in Canada, as a percent of GDP, were higher than US healthcare costs as a percent of GDP before the implementation of the Canadian single-payer system. Then, when it was fully implemented, costs dropped dramatically and decreased below those of the United States, graphically demonstrating the savings that can be realized from a single-payer system like Medicare For All. Perhaps, even more important, since adopting its plan in 1972, Canada has seen its healthcare costs rise, but at a much lower rate than the United States, as the U.S. and Canada lines diverge over nearly 50 years, demonstrating that a single-payer system not only immediately saves money as against a free market system, but also controls costs much more effectively over time. This contrast is even more pronounced because Canada does not include prescription drugs in its NHP (see Appendix), and if it did, healthcare costs would be even lower. Also, Canada's lower costs are achieved with higher quality scores than the United States (examples are in Chapter 2) as reported by the Organisation for Economic Co-operation and Development (OECD) and Commonwealth Fund in the studies identified in footnotes 2 and 3 in Chapter 2. Such a comparison clearly illustrates the cost-effectiveness of a single-payer system, like Medicare For All, versus a free market system in the United States.

Is the reduction of overhead and other costs associated with a plethora of insurance companies, as we explored in the prior chapter, the only factor in the cost-effectiveness of a single-payer system? Although it is a critical factor in cost reduction, there is another major factor at work, the national negotiating leverage with doctors, hospitals, pharmaceutical companies, and other healthcare providers.

Medicare currently pays doctors, hospital, and other providers lower fees because of its negotiating leverage, based on the number of lives it covers and plan consistency, versus that of any single insurance company. The Centers for Medicare and Medicaid Services, CMS, estimates that Medicare pays doctors a much smaller rate than what private insurers pay.[2] An article in the *New York Times* on May 10, 2019, reported on a RAND Study that showed hospitals across America paid 2.4 times Medicare rates for patients with private insurance.[3] Richard Scheffler, a health economist at the University of California Berkley, commented about the RAND study "market forces are clearly not working... prices vary widely and are two and a half times higher than Medicare payment rates without any apparent reason." And compared with current Medicare, Medicare For All would have even greater negotiating leverage. This leverage can lower costs upon implementation and, more importantly, represent a major element in cost-control in the future.

Yet, in spite of the potentially lower rates, 42% of physicians strongly support a single-payer healthcare system while 14% are somewhat supportive according to a recent Merritt Hawkins Survey of Physicians.[4] Their support can be attributed to a number of reasons, and although reimbursement for their services may be lower under Medicare For All, their administrative costs would plummet, as we observed in the chart in Chapter 3 showing that under our current free market system of private insurance, physicians' billing-related expenses are more than five times higher than under a single-payer system. So, although a doctor's fees may decrease, so will her/his expenses.

Other reasons for why doctors support Medicare For All can be illustrated in discussions the author has engaged in with doctors practicing in California and New Jersey. Their responses to the question why they like their current Medicare patients despite the lower reimbursement for their services was quite consistent and represented by the author's interview with Dr. Gary Dolowich, a physician practicing in Santa Cruz, California.[5] He knew he would get paid, no insurance company second guessing or questioning his professional judgment, much less time spent on complying with different insurance company policies, and less paperwork and time spent negotiating with insurance companies.

So, now that we have reviewed the excessive cost of our broken free market healthcare system, how much can be saved by implementing a single-payer system, or Medicare For All? A study by the University of Massachusetts, as well as one reported in the medical journal *Annals of Internal Medicine*, and a Yale Epidemiology study reported in the medical journal *Lancet* estimate savings of between $500 and $600 billion per year. (Even Charles Blahous, Sr. Research Strategist of the very conservative Mercatus Center, estimated that if private insurance rates were reduced to reflect Medicare rates, a savings of 40% would be realized.)[6] These savings are mostly achieved by eliminating the duplicative administrative and marketing costs of our profit-based insurance industry and allowing for the negotiation of medical services and pharmaceuticals on a national level. The savings for each study are shown in Table 6.1.

Table 6.1 Medicare For All annual savings

University of Massachusetts: $500 billion[7]
Yale Epidemiology, *Lancet*: $500 billion[8]
Annals of Internal Medicine: $600 billion[9]

The savings numbers above are rounded and represent three of the most expert and comprehensive studies on Medicare Savings. The dollar range is wide because, like all projections, they are based on a number of critical assumptions.

Another study by the Congressional Budget Office in 2020 reported projected national health spending to 2030 under our current healthcare system as compared with a single-payer system. Our current system was projected to spend $6.63 trillion, while a single-payer system would spend between $5.89 trillion and $6.59 trillion.[10] This would result in annual savings under a single-payer system of between $40 billion and $740 billion.

As the reader can surmise, a great deal of professional scholarly analysis is needed to determine the dollar amounts associated with the elements above. Therefore, for readers who have a greater interest, a further analysis and detailed discussion of the projections, as well as of other studies, is presented in the next section.

More Detailed Discussion of Savings Calculation

Savings Projection and Healthcare Utilization

In the first section of this chapter, cost savings projected by three major studies were presented, ranging from $500 to $600 billion annually. The overall paradigm used for these projections is as follows:

- Start with current healthcare spending
- Subtract savings from reducing insurance company overhead
- Subtract savings from reducing doctor, hospital, and other provider administrative costs
- Subtract drug price savings from bulk purchase negotiation
- Add costs of new utilization, including doctor visits and hospitalizations
- Result is new projected spending on healthcare
- Subtract projected spending from beginning spending to obtain total savings

We also discussed that depending on the estimations in each of these areas, savings projections can vary rather significantly, as can be seen in the range from $500 billion for the University of Massachusetts and Yale Epidemiology studies to $600 billion for the *Annals of Internal Medicine* study.

Each of the areas in the paradigm can differ depending on various assumptions, and we will discuss this somewhat further later in this section when we examine a study by the Urban Institute which projected a cost increase, not savings, under Medicare For All.

Here, we will more closely examine the projections of the increase in healthcare utilization, the major component of the difference in two of the studies cited above, the University of Massachusetts and the *Annals of Internal Medicine* study. Utilization overall is measured by doctor visits and in-patient hospitalizations.

The University of Massachusetts study assumes that healthcare utilization will increase by 12% when Medicare For All is implemented. The authors base their projection on a study by Brat-Goldberg that found when individuals moved from a zero-cost sharing plan to a high deductible plan, their overall utilization declined by 12–14%. However, this study presents the opposite situation from Medicare For All implementation, and therefore, may not apply, or apply to a much lesser degree. Here, individuals will feel directly monetarily penalized by having to pay more money for a plan, and since money is a powerful motivator, especially in a penalty situation, it can impede utilization rather dramatically. If Medicare For All is implemented, the analogous situation is that individuals will pay nothing if they utilize healthcare services, as opposed to directly increasing their costs. The motivation here is far less direct, involving no out-of-pocket money. This argument is supported by the author's experience designing pay and incentive plans for employees, as well as motivational theory.

More importantly than the theoretical argument presented above, the University of Massachusetts study authors openly admit in their discussion of utilization that theirs is a "high-end" estimate and that other studies, including their discussion of the "Thorpe Approach," show that utilization increases are likely to be modest, well below the 12% they use for their projections.[11]

Additionally, beyond the author's discussion, three important studies directly refute the "high-end" assumption about utilization increases made in the University of Massachusetts study. Referencing doctor utilization, a study by Gaffney, MD; McCormick, MD; Bor, MD; Woolhandler, MD; and Himmelstein, MD entitled "Utilization of Physician Care: Evidence from the 2014 Affordable Care Act and 1966 Medicare/Medicaid Expansions," in the American Journal of Public Health[12] concluded that "Past coverage expansions in the United States...have not increased society-wide utilization," and "These findings suggest that future expansions may not cause....swings in utilization." A second study examined hospital utilization, in the *Annals of Internal Medicine* of August 6, 2019, by

Gaffney, MD; McCormick, MD; Bor, MD; and Goldman, MD, entitled "The Effects on Hospital Utilization of the 1966 and 2014 Health Insurance Coverage Expansion in the United States."[13] As a prelude to their study, the authors explain that persons with comprehensive insurance use more hospital care than those who are uninsured or have high deductible plans, so analysts generally assume that expanding coverage will increase the use of in-patient hospital services. As we have seen, this is the case in the University of Massachusetts study. However, to the contrary, after a thorough examination of the date, this study concludes that past expansions were associated with little or no change in society-wide hospital use. A third study by Gaffney, MD; Woolhandler, MD; and Himmelstein, MD entitled "The Effect of Large-Scale Health Coverage Expansions in Wealthy Nations on Society-wide Healthcare Utilization," published in the *Journal of General Internal Medicine* in 2020 validated that the lack of utilization increases in the United States applied to other countries, concluding that in 13 wealthy nations studied, "Almost all (expansions) had either a small or no effect on society-wide utilization."[14]

In summary, these studies demonstrated that implementing a major expansion in healthcare coverage, like Medicare For All, will result in little, if any, increase in utilization. If we apply this to the University of Massachusetts study which projected a 12% increase in utilization, the overall cost savings approximate those of the *Annals of Internal Medicine* study at between $600 and $650 billion annually. This discussion and conclusion can also be applied to the Yale Epidemiology study.

Further, an examination of studies can easily suggest that the savings reported around $600 billion may be understated. A $600 billion annual savings projection in the study by Himmelstein et al. in the *Annals of Internal Medicine* represents savings achieved through overhead and administrative cost reductions alone.[15] Another study by the US/Canadian Pharmaceutical Working Group, "Estimated Effects of Proposed Reforms on US National Pharmaceutical Expenditures" projects a savings of over $150 billion if measures like those in Medicare For All are adopted.[16] Therefore, if savings of two studies are combined, a savings projection of over $750 billion annually can easily be projected and is certainly not out of the question.

Urban Institute and Other Projections

There have been other studies that actually project an increase in healthcare costs overall if Medicare For All is implemented. A few have been conducted by politically conservative organizations that use questionable assumptions in the elements that are components of cost/savings projections. In this section, we will use the Urban Institute's conclusion about the components of projections because the Institute tends to be a more center to left-leaning organization and, therefore, expectations were that their conclusion would show a savings. Instead, they predicted an increase in healthcare spending. We will use the Institute's study as an example of the assumptions that more conservative organizations use to project costs.[17]

The Urban Institute projects healthcare spending to increase from $52 trillion over ten years under our current system to $59 trillion over ten years if Medicare For All is implemented. That result equals an increase in healthcare spending of about $700 billion per year. This is in marked contrast to the three studies we have discussed in this book that project a savings of between $500 and $600 billion annually. So, why the discrepancy? The answer lies in the assumptions used in the components of the projections explained previously as outlined at the beginning of this section. Again, they are:

- Start with current healthcare spending
- Subtract savings from reducing insurance company overhead
- Subtract savings from reducing doctor, hospital, and other provider administrative costs
- Subtract drug price savings from bulk purchase negotiation
- Add costs of new utilization, including doctor visits and hospitalizations. The result is new projected spending on healthcare
- Subtract projected spending from beginning spending to obtain total savings

We will begin our examination with savings on insurance company overhead. The Urban Institute assumed minimal savings because they assumed overhead under Medicare For All would be 6%. In fact, overhead costs in Canada, with a single-payer system similar to Medicare For All, and Medicare in the United States are both at around 2%. So, the Urban Institute projected overhead costs under Medicare For All at three times what would actually be expected, and these savings are quite large in dollar terms as we have discussed previously in this book. Second, the Urban Institute excluded savings on doctors' and hospitals' administrative costs which we have shown to be substantial. Lastly, the Urban Institute projected a utilization surge of nearly 21%, a dramatic increase over the University of Massachusetts' 12%, which we have explained in the beginning of this chapter appears to be excessive.

So, the reader can readily understand that the combination of the assumptions explained above result in the Urban Institute (and some other conservative authored studies) projections of cost increases under Medicare For All. Based on the information explored in this book, those assumptions appear to be in conflict with research, actual data, and experience.

Other Potential Savings

In this section, we will explore other potential savings not quantified in the studies discussed in the prior two sections.

A single-payer system will reduce the high cost of care for those uninsured citizens using hospital emergency rooms for their healthcare. Under the Emergency Medical Treatment & Labor Act (EMTALA) of 1980, public and community hospitals are forbidden to deny care to anyone. As a result, many uninsured and underinsured individuals visit emergency rooms of these hospitals to provide basic healthcare for colds, insomnia, rashes, etc. By facilitating these patients to visit private doctor's offices instead of the very high cost and expensive emergency room venue, Medicare For All can save even more money.

A single-payer system can provide additional savings by emphasizing evidence-based medicine, quality of care, preventive care, and improved health outcomes, versus our current free market insurance company-driven method of fee-for service. Additionally, many studies have shown that health insurance plan copays and deductibles cause people to delay or even neglect care. A 2018 Commonwealth Fund International Health Policy Survey reported that 40% of Americans skipped seeing a doctor because of cost.[18] And a study by Harvard reported in early 2018 in the *Journal of Clinical Oncology* that woman in high deductible plans delayed getting care, even though early treatment is key in cancer care.[19] That percent was much lower in other countries. Overall, Medicare For All could facilitate a move away from the current emphasis on treating sickness and more toward ensuring health though early treatment.

Another example is exercise. The *New York Times* reported a study which estimated that lack of exercise drives at least $117 billion in annual healthcare spending in the United States.[20] Researchers at the National Cancer Institute and the Centers for Disease Control and Prevention (CDC) published a report in *BMJ Open Sport and Exercise Medicine* in February 2021 showing that for those who exercised moderately throughout their adult lives, a savings of $1,350 in healthcare costs was realized.[20] Yet, despite these savings, more than half of the American adult population is sedentary. Health coaches working from the lead of doctors have been very successful in helping people in developing and adhering to an exercise program. Health coaches provide patients with the knowledge, tools, skills, motivation, and confidence to be successful in their own care in the areas of exercise, nutrition, pharmaceutical compliance, and behavioral health, among other areas. A study by the University of Southern Main found patients helped by health coaches saved $412 a month in healthcare expenses per patient.[21] This type of approach to healthcare is not popular and is difficult to institute under our current for-profit system but would be a natural extension of Medicare For All.

By eliminating cost of care in patient access to care, Medicare For All would foster disease management, preventive care, and early disease intervention which would save money by avoiding more expensive care like hospitalizations, surgery, and intensive care for diseases such as diabetes, asthma, hypertension, and cancer as they progress. A study by Baicker et al. in the *Quarterly Journal of Economics* entitled "Behavioral Hazard to Health Insurance," stated, "Creating cost barriers to treatment at any given time can lead to increased overall health care costs because consumers are not receiving preventive treatments...."[22]

With respect to medication, the pharmaceutical industry has known for some time, based on their medication adherence tracking data, that increased costs leads to non-adherence, with patients either not filling their prescriptions and/or delaying taking their medication. This was confirmed by a study published in an article by Aina Abell in *Adherence*.[23] This too can easily lead to high costs as diseases progress in severity without medication, causing the need for more intensive and expensive treatment.

Also, Medicare For All would establish a national healthcare treatment database, allowing for greater development of evidence-based medicine by extracting and analyzing information from the database to firmly establish which medical treatments are most effective. Treating patients more effectively, efficiently, and certainly curing patients would have an impact on driving down costs.

Additionally, unpublished research that the author has spearheaded shows that Medicare For All would lower costs for businesses by reducing absenteeism and increasing labor productivity gained through a healthier workforce.[24] These gains would be achieved by employers at the same time their burden of providing healthcare coverage for employees was eliminated. Lowering operating costs would aid American industry's competitiveness in today's global environment.

Reference List

1 As reported by Physicians for a National Health Program, Short Slide Deck, 2019.
2 How do Medicare Physician Fees Compare with Private Payers? By Mark E. Miller, Stephen Zuckerman, and Michael Gates, National Institutes of Health US National Library of Medicine, https://www.ncbi.nlm.nih.gov/pmc/articles/PMC4193371/.
3 Many Hospitals Charge Double or Even Triple What Medicare Would Pay, by Reed Abelson, *NY Times*, May 9, 2019, https://www.nytimes.com/2019/05/09/health/hospitals-prices-medicare.html.
4 Merritt Hawkins Survey, Survey: 42% of Physicians Strongly Support Single Payer Healthcare, 35% Strongly Oppose, Aug 14, 2017, https://www.

merritthawkins.com/uploadedFiles/mha_singlepayer_press_release_2017(1).pdf.

5 Ken Lefkowitz interview with Gary Dolowich, a physician in Santa Cruz, California, Dec 12, 2019.

6 The Costs of a National Single-Payer Healthcare System, by Charles Blahous, Mercatus Center at George Mason University, Arlington, VA, July 2018. https://www.mercatus.org/system/files/blahous-costs-medicare-mercatus-working-paper-vl_1.pdf.

7 University of Massachusetts (R. Pollin et al., Economic analysis of Medicare For All, Political Economic Research Institute (PERI) UMass Amherst, Dec 3, 2018, https://peri.umass.edu/publication/item/1127-economic-analysis-of-medicare-for-all).

8 Yale Epidemiology (Galvani et al., Improving the Prognosis of Health Care in the USA, Lancet, Feb. 15, 2020).

9 Annals of Internal Medicine study (Himmelstein et al., Health Care Costs in the US and Canada, 2017, *Annals of Internal Medicine*, Jan, 2020. Doi: 10.7326/M19-2818).

10 How CBO Analyzes the Costs of Proposals for Single-Payer Health Care Systems That Are Based on Medicare's Fee-for-Service Program: Working Paper 2020-08, Dec 10, 2020, 56811-Data-Underlying-Exhibits, Exhibit 1.1 Spreadsheet, first four options, https://www.cbo.gov/publication/56811.

11 Reviewer Assessments of Economic Analysis of Medicare For All, University of Massachusetts Political Economy Institute, by Robert Pollin, James Heintz, Peter Arno, Jeannette Wicks-Lin, and Michael Ash, Sept 2017, https://peri.umass.edu/reviewer-assessments-of-economic-analysis-of-medicare-for-all#woolhandlerl.

12 Utilization of Physician Care: Evidence from the 2014 Affordable Care Act and 1966 Medicare/Medicaid Expansions, by Adam Gaffney, Danny McCormick, David Bor, Steffie Woolhandler, and David Himmelstein, *American Journal of Public Health*, Dec 2109, https://ajph.aphapublications.org/page/authors.html.

13 The Effects on Hospital Utilization of the 1966 and 2014 Health Insurance Coverage Expansions in the United States, by Adam Gaffney, Danny McCormick, David Borr, Anna Goldman, Steffie Woolhandler, and David Himmelstein, *Annals of Internal Medicine*, Aug 6, 2019, https://www.acpjournals.org/doi/full/10.7326/M18-2806.

14 The Effect of Large-scale Health Coverage Expansions in Wealthy Nations on Society-Wide Healthcare Utilization, by Adam Gaffney, Steffie Woolhandler, and David Himmelstein, *Journal of General Internal Medicine*, Aug 2020, National Library of Medicine, CDC, NIH, https://pubmed.ncbi.nlm.nih.gov/31745857/.

15 Health Care Administrative costs in the United States and Canada, 2017, by David U. Himmelstien, Terry Campbell, Steffie Woolhandler, *Annals of Internal Medicine, Medicine and Public Issues*, Jan 21, 2020, https://www.acp-journals.org/doi/abs/10.7326/m19-2818.

16 Estimated Effects of Proposed Reforms on US National Pharmaceutical Expenditures the US/Canadian Pharmaceutical Working Group, www.pnhp.org/sites/default/files/Pharma_Table7_pdf; www.googlesearch?q=the+US%2FCanadian+Pharmaceutical+Working+Group%2C+"Estimated+Effects+of+Proposed+Reforms+on+US+National+Pharmaceutical+Expenditures+&tbm=isch&ved=2ahUKEwiYlvPs3LbzA.

17 The Urban Institute's Attack on Single Payer: Ridiculous Assumptions Yield Ridiculous Estimates, David Himmelstein and Clare Fauke, *Huffington*

Post, May 9, 2016, 7:31 EDT. 05/09/2016 07:31 pm ET Updated, May 10, 2017, https://www.huffpost.com/entry/the-urban-institutes-attack-on-single-payer-ridiculous-assumptions-yield-ridiculous-estimates_b_9876640.

18 Health Insurance Coverage Eight Years after the ACA: Fewer Uninsured Americans and Shorter Coverage Gaps, But More Underinsured Sara R. Collins Vice President The Commonwealth Fund, by Sara R. Collins, Herman K. Bhupal, and Micelle M. Day, Feb 2019, https://www.commonwealthfund.org/sites/default/files/2019-02/Collins_hlt_ins_coverage_8_years_after_ACA_2018_biennial_survey_sb.pdf.

19 Women in High Deductible Plans Delayed Getting Care, *Journal of Clinical Oncology*, www.google.com/search?q=Journal+of+Clinical+Oncology+that+woman+in+high+deductible+plans+delayed+getting+care%2C+&tbm.

20 Lifelong Exercise Adds Up to Big Health Care Savings, by Gretchen Reynolds, *The NY Times*, June 16, 2021, https://www.nytimes.com/2021/06/16/well/move/exercise-health-care-cost-savings.html.

21 We Could All Use a Health Coach, by Jane E. Brody, *The New York Times*, June 7, 2021, https://www.nytimes.com/2021/06/07/well/live/health-coach-benefits.html.

22 Behavioral Hazard in Health Insurance, by Katherine Baicker, Sendhil Mullainathan, and Joshua Schwartstein, *Quarterly Journal of Economics*, 130(4), https://www.hbs.edu/ris/Publication%20Files/Behavioral%20Hazard%20in%20Health%20Insurance_141863a4-c31b-4f78-b358-2bb32db169b5.pdf.

23 Medication Adherence Suffers Because of High Drug Costs, by Aina Abell, *Adherence*, 26(4), P29, Apr 2020, https://www.pharmacytoday.org/article/S1042-0991(20)30300-5/fulltext.

24 Author's research while working at AstraZeneca Corporation as US Director of Benefits, 2015–2018.

7 The ACA and Other Issues

The Affordable Care Act, a Public Option, and Other Recent Improvements

The Affordable Care Act, or ACA, commonly known as Obamacare, signed into law in March 2010, included many needed healthcare reforms. Examples are precluding insurance companies from considering preexisting conditions in coverage consideration and pricing, expanding the Medicaid program, and offering subsidies for lower income individuals in the insurance exchange networks that it established. However, the ACA left our broken free market healthcare system in place, did not save money, did not establish a system for controlling healthcare costs in the future, and did not provide for universal coverage, all of which are addressed by Medicare For All.

The current Biden administration prefers expanding the ACA by offering a public option in addition to the coverage offered by insurance companies, presumably with a lower price tag for consumers. Unfortunately, such a program would not lower healthcare costs, but in fact increase them, by about $700 billion annually according to statements made by Mr. Biden.[1]

Cost is just one issue surrounding the idea of a public option. The rational for the plan, as outlined by the President, is based on his perceived need to protect employer-based plans since his belief is that employees do not want them eliminated as they would be under Medicare For All.[1] However, this position is based on a stale viewpoint and old data when employer-based plans provided comprehensive coverage at little or no cost to employees. In fact, many of these plans, especially offered by larger employers, were referred to as "Cadillac" plans. Circumstances have changed rather dramatically over the past few years, however, as most employers have found the increasing economic burden of providing healthcare plans a drain on profits and have increased premiums, deductibles, and copays substantially. As indicated previously, a 2020 Kaiser Family Foundation Survey reported that the average amount an employee pays for his/her healthcare coverage averages about $5,600 a year with an average deductible of nearly $1,650 annually.[2] And this does

DOI: 10.4324/9781003286271-7

not include increasing copays. Hardly a healthcare plan to covet despite what supporters of a public option contend.

Also, a public option would cost more than its supporters estimate because of the concept of adverse selection. If the public option was priced lower than private insurance, it would attract a sicker and more expensive population. That's adverse selection. This could easily make the public option unsustainable from a cost perspective. In fact, under the ACA, healthcare cooperatives were established which tended to offer lower copays under their plans. The result was that, overall, they attracted a sicker, higher cost population, and nearly all of them failed because of that as well as other factors.

Another position relative to a public option is that it represents a transition toward Medicare For All. This is also a flawed concept. Moving directly to Medicare For All would be a managed, controlled process, far preferable and efficient than a haphazard and uncontrolled process that would result from hoping that a public option would be a transition to Medicare For All. Additionally, the longer the transition period, the longer the lost opportunity for cost savings continues, and the longer the society condones leaving individuals with no healthcare coverage.

During the first half year of the Biden Administration, a number of improvements in the ACA have been introduced. Subsidies provided by the government have been expanded. To address COVID-related issues, the open enrollment period has been lengthened, the federal government will pay the entire premium for coverage under the Consolidated Omnibus Budget Reconciliation Act (COBRA) for those whose have lost their jobs or had their work hours reduced by their employer, and for those who experienced unemployment, they are eligible for free premiums on certain plans offered under the ACA. Also, under consideration is lowering Medicare eligibility age to 60, expansion of Medicare to include vision, hearing, and dental, allowing Medicare to negotiate drug prices, and implementing an out-of-pocket cap.

Additionally, the Biden Administration has proposed importing prescription drugs from Canada in order to lower costs. It is questionable whether this type of effort is workable and can actually be implemented. The Biden Administration also issued rules to protect patients against "surprise billing" for out of network services. While quite commendable, their impact on medical costs will most certainly be diluted. This is because health insurers' networks are negotiated so the insurer can save costs in our free market, for-profit healthcare system. Therefore, we can expect that to counter the cost savings lost by insurers under the new rules, they will turn to another avenue to make up for the reduced profits, such as increasing premiums for coverage. Under a free market system, trying to control costs is like squeezing a balloon – when you squeeze it one place, it pops out in another. This is humorously pointed out in the comic strip "Pearls Before Swine" printed in the *Philadelphia Inquirer* newspaper (Figure 7.1).[3]

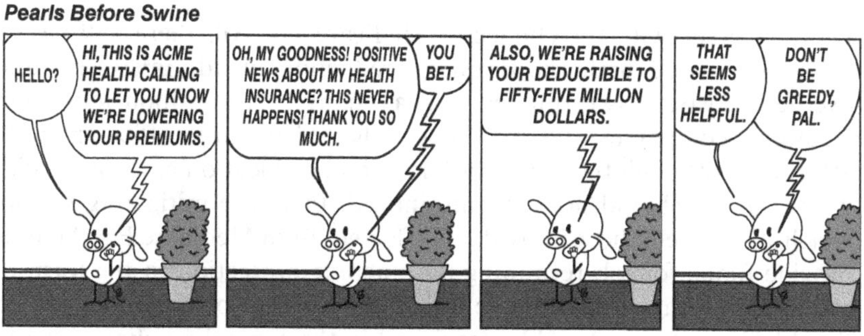

Pearls Before Swine

Figure 7.1 Humorous cartoon from the *Philadelphia Inquirer*

All of these efforts by the Biden Administration outlined above highlight the fact that our free market system simply just doesn't work. Clearly, it's time to stop tweaking our current system and implement Medicare For All, the cost-effective single-payer approach.

Current Government Spending on Healthcare

Research by Himmelstein and Woolhandler, published in the *American Journal of Public Health* entitled "The Current and Projected Taxpayer Share of US Health Costs," calculated that 64% of healthcare spending is already publicly funded and will grow to over 67% by 2024.[4] This includes spending for Medicare, Medicaid, Veterans Affairs, coverage for government employees, and tax subsidies for company-provided plans through employers' tax deductions for employee healthcare coverage. Unfortunately, although some of the components do have lower administrative costs and pricing, in the aggregate, they keep our current broken free market system in place, and they all lack the overall negotiating leverage of a national plan. So, the question can easily be posed, why not realize the entire savings and gain the full negotiating leverage by including the other 36% of spending through Medicare For All?

Support for Medicare For All

Three polls by major research organizations, the Pew Research Center, the Kaiser Family Foundation, and Gallup Inc., report that about 60% of Americans support the federal government providing healthcare to all residents through a single-payer system.[2] Additionally, a Merritt Hawkins Survey of Physicians revealed that about 55% of physicians support a single-payer system like Medicare For All (see Chapter 6). These studies indicate strong support for the implementation of Medicare For All already exists.

Insurance Industry/Other Job Loss

Unfortunately, with the change to Medicare For All, there will be job losses associated with the dramatic reduction in administrative and overhead costs. It is estimated that as many as 1.8 million jobs from insurance companies and from hospitals and doctors' offices may be affected.[5] Although the pain of job loss, and dislocation associated with it, is real and should never be minimized, there are mitigating factors which should help those individuals affected. Both Medicare For All bills provide funds for job retraining and income protection in the form of extended severance pay for the individuals losing jobs. Quite a few of those losing jobs may well be employed in the expanding clinical workforce under Medicare For All. In a more general economic perspective, lower healthcare spending nationally will stimulate the economy as will companies being relieved of the burden of providing healthcare, resulting in rising employment overall. Individuals suffering job loss, especially those retrained, may very well find employment as a result.

Other perspectives are helpful in understanding the magnitude of the job loss, but of course, not particularly helpful on an individual level for those actually losing jobs. Each year in the United States, there are tens of millions job separations consisting of layoffs, quits, and firings. The 1.8 million estimated job losses associated with Medicare For All implementation is but a fraction of annual job separations and, within that context on a macro level, doesn't quite appear as severe as the absolute number. Another frame of reference is the effects of technological advancements on jobs. Some four million jobs are expected to be lost in the trucking industry with the advent of self-driving vehicles,[6] and few of the individuals affected will receive federal government-funded job retraining or extended severance pay.

Funding Medicare For All

The concept of funding is used here, not paying for, because, in fact, we all pay for the overall cost of healthcare. The central issue is whether it is the insurance industry or the government that operates as the intermediate in collecting the money and paying the bills. Also, the savings already discussed in Chapter 6 will be sufficient to pay for the additional healthcare coverage provided under Medicare For All. So, there is no overall increase in healthcare spending and, as has been also discussed, Medicare For All will establish a system for controlling healthcare costs in the future. Another way to express this is that the federal government increases its share of the healthcare cost pie, but the pie shrinks. A complete exploration of the issue of funding is beyond the scope of this book since much of the issue does not fall in the realm of data analysis, but rather in the political sphere. Yet, a brief review of how the federal government might fund Medicare For All is appropriate.

There are a number of sources of funding. First, some sources of funds will occur naturally as part of Medicare For All implementation. These consist of the federal government revenue gain as both employers and individual will no longer have tax deductions for medical care. Second, employers will be relieved of providing healthcare for their employees, in an amount approximately equal to $700 billion per year. So, the government might establish an Employer Medical Contribution, or an outright tax on employers to recover some of this money. Third, could be the elimination of the Trump administration's tax cuts for higher income individuals. Fourth, a 35% minimum tax on foreign corporate earnings could be implemented, closing a very unpopular corporate tax loophole with the American public. Fifth, a change in the depreciation schedule for company investments. Sixth, an increase in the capital gains tax. And a special tax on the top 1% might also be implemented, as well as a wealth tax.

Another avenue for raising funds is to increase the Internal Revenue Service's (IRS) enforcement. The *New York Times* of April 14, 2021, reported that Charles Retting, the IRS commissioner, testified before a Senate Finance Committee hearing that if the IRS were allowed the workforce it needed to enforce the code fully, an additional $1 trillion could be collected annually.[7]

Some of these have been proposed by Senators Elizabeth Warren and Bernie Sanders as part of their support for Medicare For All. Certainly, not all of these approaches will be needed, and the ultimate decision on how to address the funding shift in implementing Medicare For All will be determined in the political arena.

Reference List

1 Statements made by President Biden during the Democratic Presidential Debate, 2020, and in numerous public speeches before and after becoming President.
2 Kaiser Family Foundation 2020 Employer Health Benefits Survey, Published: Oct 8, 2020, https://www.kff.org/health-costs/report/2020-employer-health-benefits-survey/.
3 Pearls Before Swine, printed in the Jul 21, 2021 in the Philadelphia Inquirer Newspaper Comics Section, Page C5.
4 US National Library of Medicine, National Institute of Health. https://www.ncbi.nlm.nih.gov/pmc/articles/PMC4880216/; The Current and Projected Taxpayer Shares of US Health Costs, by David Himmelstein and Steffie Woolhandler, *American Journal of Public Health*, March 2016, 106(3), 449–452. Doi: 10.2105/AJPH.2015.302997.

5 Medicare For All's Jobs Problems, by Rochana Pradham, Politico, *The Agenda*, Nov 25, 2019, 5:08 EST, https://www.politico.com/news/agenda/2019/11/25/medicare-for-all-jobs-067781.
6 Stick Shift, Autonomous Vehicles, Driving Jobs, and the Future of Work, Algernon Austin Demos, Cherrie Bucknor Center for Economic and Policy Research, Kevin Cashman Center for Economic and Policy Research, and Maya Rockeymore Center for Global Policy Solutions Center for Global Policy Solutions. Washington, DC.
7 The U.S. Is Losing $1 Trillion Annually to Tax Cheats, by Alan Rappeport, *The NY Times*, April 13, 2021, Updated Sept 8, 2021, https://www.nytimes.com/live/2021/04/13/business/stock-market-today.

8 Summary

After the information and data presented in the first seven chapters, it is appropriate to present a brief summary of the practical and economic benefits of implementing Medicare For All. Of course, these advantages are in addition to the marked advantages of Medicare For All in addressing social, humanitarian, ethical, and equity issues and concerns.

Economic/practical benefits of Medicare For All:

- Fixes America's currently broken free market system
- Removes layers of complexity, overhead, and confusion
- Saves at least $500–$600 billion a year
- Addresses runaway healthcare costs by establishing a cost management structure for the future
- Allows doctors and other healthcare providers to focus on patients, not administrative issues, saving money and time
- Builds on Medicare, a successful, popular, efficient, and reliable program working for over 50 years. A base underlying structure is already in place, meaning no massive overall design and infrastructure construction is required.

DOI: 10.4324/9781003286271-8

Appendix

The Canadian and German Healthcare Systems

The Canadian Healthcare System

Periodically, we have referred to the Canadian healthcare system as a yardstick, and at times, a point of reference. Therefore, for the reader's edification, it is important to provide an overall understanding of the Canadian system. The following is a summary of key aspects of the Canadian healthcare system. The information source is the detailed description outlined on the Canadian Government's website.[1]

The publicly funded healthcare system provides for access to a broad range of healthcare services. Canadians refer to the system as "Medicare." It is best described overall as an interlocking set of ten provincial and three territorial health systems. The system is funded through the national government and administered by the Provinces which are roughly equivalent to states in America.

The Canadian healthcare system is financed with general revenue raised through federal, provincial, and territorial taxation. This includes personal and corporate taxes, sales taxes, payroll levies, and other revenue. Provinces can also charge a health premium on their residents to help pay for publicly funded healthcare services. However, non-payment of one of these premiums is not allowed to limit access to medically necessary health services.

An important point is that most doctors work in independent or group practices and are not employed by the government. Some work in community health centers, hospital-based group practices, primary healthcare teams, or are affiliated with hospital out-patient departments. Nurses are primarily employed in acute care institutions (hospitals); however, they also provide community healthcare, including home care and public health services.

There are five key principles of the Canada Health Act:

1   Public Administration: The provincial and territorial plans must be administered and operated on a non-profit basis by a public authority accountable to the provincial or territorial government.

2   Comprehensiveness: The provincial and territorial plans must insure all medically necessary services provided by hospitals, medical practitioners, and dentists working within a hospital setting.
3   Universality: The provincial and territorial plans must entitle all insured persons to health insurance coverage on uniform terms and conditions.
4   Accessibility: The provincial and territorial plans must provide all insured persons reasonable access to medically necessary hospital and physician services without financial or other barriers.
5   Portability: The provincial and territorial plans must cover all insured persons when they move to another province or territory within Canada and when they travel abroad. The provinces and territories have some limits on coverage for services provided outside Canada and may require prior approval for non-emergency services delivered outside their jurisdiction.

The federal government's roles in the healthcare system include setting and administering national principles under the Canada Health Act and financial support to the provinces and territories. Other functions, including funding and/or delivery of primary and supplementary services to certain groups of people including: First Nations people living on reserves; Inuit; serving members of the Canadian Armed Forces; eligible veterans; inmates in federal penitentiaries; and some groups of refugee claimants.

Direct federal delivery of services to First Nations people and Inuit includes primary care and emergency services on remote and difficult to access reserves where no provincial or territorial services are readily available; community-based health programs both on reserves and in Inuit communities; and a non-insured health benefits program (drug, dental, and ancillary health services) for First Nations people and Inuit living anywhere within the borders of Canada. These services are provided mostly at health centers, nursing stations, in-patient treatment centers, and through community health promotion programs. Government and Aboriginal organizations are increasingly working together to integrate the delivery of these services with the provincial and territorial systems.

The federal government is also responsible for health protection and regulation (e.g., regulation of pharmaceuticals, food, and medical devices), consumer safety, and disease surveillance and prevention. It also provides support for health promotion and health research. In addition, the federal government has instituted health-related tax measures, including tax credits for medical expenses, disability, caregivers and infirm dependents; tax rebates to public institutions for health services; and deductions for private health insurance premiums for the self-employed.

The Canada Health Act establishes criteria and conditions for health insurance plans that must be met by provinces and territories in order for them to receive full federal cash transfers in support of health. Provinces and territories are required to provide reasonable access to medically necessary hospital and doctors' services.

The provinces and territories administer and deliver most of Canada's healthcare services, with all provincial and territorial health insurance plans expected to meet national principles established under the Canada Health Act. Each provincial and territorial health insurance plan covers medically necessary hospital and doctors' services that are provided on a pre-paid basis, without direct charges at the point of service. The provincial and territorial governments fund these services with assistance from federal cash and tax transfers.

The roles of the provincial and territorial governments in healthcare include:

• Administration of the health insurance plan;
• Planning and funding of care in hospitals and other health facilities;
• Services provided by doctors and other health professionals;
• Planning and implementation of health promotion and public health initiatives;
• Negotiation of fee schedules with health professionals.

Additional health services are provided by the provinces and territories to certain groups like low-income residents, seniors, and children that are not generally covered under the publicly funded healthcare system. These supplementary health benefits often include prescription drugs outside hospitals (prescription drugs are not part of the nationally funded system as discussed later), dental care, vision care, medical equipment and appliances like prostheses and wheelchairs, as well as the services of other health professionals such as physiotherapists.

The first point of contact within the system is primary healthcare services provided by primary care physicians. Primary care physicians represent the anchors of the healthcare system, providing two key functions. First, they are the deliverers of first-contact healthcare services. Second, they also coordinate a patients' healthcare services. This is done for two reasons: to ensure continuity of care and to facilitate services across the healthcare system when more specialized care is needed, as from specialist providers or in hospitals, for example.

Primary healthcare services have become increasingly comprehensive and may include prevention and treatment of common diseases and injuries; basic emergency services; referrals to and coordination with other levels of care, such as hospital and specialist care; primary mental healthcare; palliative and end-of-life care; health promotion; healthy child development; primary maternity care; and rehabilitation services.

When necessary, patients who require further diagnosis or treatment are referred to other healthcare services, like diagnostic testing, and healthcare professionals, such as physician specialists, nurse practitioners, and allied health professionals other than physicians and nurses.

In secondary services after primary care, a patient may be referred for specialized care at a hospital, at a long-term care facility or in the community. The majority of Canadian hospitals are operated by community boards of trustees, voluntary organizations, or regional health authorities established by provincial/territorial governments. Hospitals are generally funded through annual, global budgets that set overall expenditure targets or limits (as opposed to fee-for-service arrangements, as in the United States) negotiated with the provincial and territorial ministries of health, or with a regional health authority or board. Global funding is the principal approach for hospital reimbursement in Canada, although a number of provinces have experimented with supplementary funding approaches.

Secondary healthcare services are also provided in the home or community and in long-term and chronic care institutions. Referrals to home, community, or institutional care can be made by doctors, hospitals, community agencies, families, and patients themselves. Patient needs are assessed by medical professionals, and services are coordinated to provide continuity of care. Care is provided by a range of formal, informal, and volunteer caregivers.

Recent reforms focused on primary healthcare delivery, including setting up more community primary healthcare centers that provide on-call services around-the-clock; creating primary healthcare teams; placing greater emphasis on promoting health, preventing illness and injury, and managing chronic diseases; increasing coordination and integration of comprehensive health services; and improving the work environments of primary healthcare providers.

After providing this summary description of the Canadian healthcare system for the reader's understanding, it is important to review two key issues associated with Canadian healthcare: wait times and pharmaceutical coverage.

Wait Times

One of the most controversial issues within the Canadian system is wait times, which tend to be longer than those in many other countries, including the United States. This is a complex issue with many aspects which we will discuss.

First and foremost is the fact that it is not the single-payer system that causes the longer wait times, as discussed in an article by Aaron. E. Carroll, M.D., M.S. "Five Myths About Canadian Health Care," published by AARP,[2] Dr. Carroll states, "The wait times that Canada might experience are not caused by its being a single-payer system." "Our (the United States) single-payer system, which is called Medicare manages not to have the "wait times" issue that Canada's does. There must, therefore, be some other reason for the wait times."

There are, in fact, a number of reasons, but before we explore them, it is important to understand some of the nuances of Canadian wait times. In a 2018 Commonwealth Fund podcast interview,[3] chief medical information officer at an academic and research healthcare organization in Canada, Christopher Hayes, provided some insights about wait times.

Dr. Hayes states in the interview:

> It depends on what do you think you're waiting for. So, if you are in a hospital and you need surgery you don't wait. It gets done in – if it needs to be done in 30 minutes it will be done in 30 minutes. If you need an MRI for care provided in a hospital you will get it whenever – depending on where you are because not every hospital has an MRI, but you will be prioritized and that will happen probably as quickly as it can be done anywhere. It is as the priority drops or is deemed less by whomever that the wait – so the waits are how long will you wait to see a specialist after seeing your family doctor. I mean, the one that people will talk about is cataracts, hip surgeries, non – not cancer type surgeries, where there – things will get worse if you don't get treated. And so you can wait months for those surgeries.

So, in Canada, the wait time is influenced by the relative need and disease severity of the person being treated and according to the availability of services in the area.

With this understanding, we can return to the causes of wait times. Many experts point to inefficiencies and confusion caused by federal funding with local administration which is not the case under a nationally administered system like American Medicare. This would be the same under Medicare For All. Other experts have identified a shortage of some specialists and sophisticated testing equipment, and that shortage differs by province, resulting in differences in wait times. So, in Canada, because of local administration, wait times differ widely by province. For example, to get a computed tomography (CT) scan, for the average patient in Alberta, the wait is 2.5 weeks, similar to that in the United States. While the wait for the average patient in Saskatchewan, for the same CT scan is seven weeks.

The *Journal of the College of Family Physicians of Canada* identified several factors as contributing to the wait times for access to specialists in Canada, including limited specialty care resources, inconsistency in family physicians' abilities to order advanced diagnostic tests, and higher demands on the healthcare system at large. A policy statement by the Canadian Medical Association highlighted a few changes that would reduce wait times and that should be adopted throughout the country, such as improved communication between providers and streamlining patient flow from primary to specialty care. Of course, as in any complex system, modest increased spending on some carefully studied and targeted areas would help reduce wait times.

And yet, despite the longer waits, a poll conducted by the Toronto-based Nanos Research reveals that 86.2% of Canadians overwhelmingly support strengthening public healthcare rather than expanding into for-profit services. Nik Nanos, president of Nanos Research, said of the study, "With more than 8 in 10 Canadians supporting public solutions to make public healthcare stronger, there is compelling evidence that Canadians across all demographics would prefer a public over a for-profit health care system."[4]

Additionally, a report issued by the Canadian Government, "Healthy Canadians – A Federal Report on Comparable Health Indicators," found that most Canadians, 85.2% aged 15 years and older, reported being satisfied with the way overall healthcare services were provided.[5]

Prescription Drugs

Next, we will turn to the issue of prescription drugs. The data and factual information presented here about pharmaceutical coverage in Canada have been gleaned from three major sources: an article in the *Journal of Pharmaceutical Policy and Practice* entitled "Prescription drug coverage in Canada: a review of the economic, policy and political considerations for universal pharmacare,"[6] a report in the February 2020 edition of *Health Affairs* concerning pharmaceutical coverage in Canada,[7] and a Reuters 2019 report by Kelsey Johnson and Allison Martell entitled "Canadian Panel Calls for Universal Public Drug Coverage."[8]

Canada's system of government-funded universal health insurance for medical and hospital care publicly finances nearly 100% of all expenditures for physician services and hospital care. Yet, in stark contrast, only 42% of total prescription drug expenditures are financed by government public programs. The remaining prescription drug expenditures in Canada are financed through other means. Private insurance plans finance 35% while 23% is paid out-of-pocket by patients. Approximately two-thirds of Canadian workers have private insurance coverage mostly provided by their employers. Of those citizens who have private prescription drug insurance, 17% have fixed copays and 67% pay co-insurance.

In contrast with the universal Medicare system, Canada's system of pharmaceutical coverage is a complex and largely uncoordinated mix of public and private insurance plans that differ in terms of eligibility, patient charges, coverage, and formularies. There are no national standards for public drug programs, but each province may offer some form of public subsidy for prescription drugs. Most, but not all, provinces offer the general population coverage against catastrophic costs that exceed deductibles and are established as a percentage of household income. These percentages of household income used to define deductibles vary considerably across provinces that do offer these catastrophic coverage programs. After a deductible limit is met, the government pays for all or a significant portion of the cost for eligible drug products.

Overall, this patchwork system of private and public prescription drug coverage in Canada leaves approximately one in five Canadians without coverage. Several surveys have revealed that approximately one in ten Canadian patients do not fill prescriptions written for them as a consequence of out-of-pocket costs and their inability to afford them. This should sound familiar to the reader, as the same issues exist in the United States because of the lack of coverage.

Canada is the only high-income country with a universal health insurance system that does not provide universal coverage of prescription drugs. Its fragmented and decentralized pharmaceutical coverage consists of more than 1,000 public and 100,000 private plans. This makes it challenging and difficult for smaller payers to negotiate discounts with pharmaceutical companies. Again, the same issues facing the decentralized free market system in America.

Over the past 30 years, total prescription drug spending in Canada has grown at an average annual rate of 8.1% while physician expenditures have grown at an average annual increase of 5.6%, and hospital spending increased at 4.4%. In 2017, pharmaceutical costs grew by 5.5%. In contrast, physician costs increased by 4.4% and hospital spending grew 2.9%. These differences in these increases demonstrate the power of a national single-payer system in controlling costs.

It is mostly the uncoordinated patchwork of prescription drug financing that has resulted in less favorable conditions for controlling drug spending than are found in other high-income countries with universal drug coverage. For example, total per capita expenditure on prescription drugs in Canada during 2015 was 43% greater than the average for the Organization for Economic Cooperation and Development (OECD) countries. Only the United States and Switzerland with multi-payer systems were higher. And that is despite the fact that Canada has a younger population than some of the OECD countries, like Sweden, the United Kingdom, Netherlands, and France and yet spends more per capita on pharmaceuticals than these countries. Other research has shown that consolidated coordinated prescription drug financing systems wield greater purchasing power in price negotiations with pharmaceutical companies. Therefore, they are able to achieve lower prescription drug expenditures through lower prices and more cost-conscious prescribing patterns.

National commissions have repeatedly recommended that universal prescription drug coverage, or universal pharmacare as it is often referred to in Canada, be part of Canada's universal public health insurance system. If this type of single-payer system for prescription drugs with a national formulary were to be implemented, it would provide for much greater administrative efficiency and significant purchasing power, leading to substantial cost savings. In 2017, Canada's Parliamentary Budget Officer estimated net annual cost savings of $4.2 billion annually, or approximately 17% if prescription drug coverage was included under the national healthcare program as a universal pharmacare plan. And these estimated savings take into account increased utilization. The Parliamentary Budget Officer estimated there would be more than 50 million additional prescriptions filled in Canada under a universal pharmacare program.

Physicians' support for such a program has been from the members of Canadian Doctors for Medicare. It has actively campaigned for universal pharmacare because it would save money through bulk purchasing, reduce administrative burden on physicians, increase access to medicines, and improve patient outcomes. The Canadian Federation of Nurses Unions has also campaigned for universal pharmacare, based on the same arguments made by the Canadian Doctors for Medicare.

The German Healthcare System

As the German system of healthcare was referred to in the section on the comparison with other countries' healthcare costs in Chapter 2, it is important to provide a more detailed description of the German system. The information and details in this section were referenced from a June 6, 2020, article by Miriam Blümel and Reinhard Busse, Department of Health Care Management, *Technische Universität Berlin*, which can be found on the Commonwealth Fund website.[9]

Health insurance in Germany consists of two subsystems. First is the statutory health insurance system, or SHI, consisting of sickness funds. These are not-for-profit, competing, non-government health insurance plans. Second is private health insurance. Long-term care services are covered separately under Germany's mandatory, statutory long-term care insurance, or LTCI. Universal health insurance is mandatory in Germany. The statutory health insurance provides for out-patient, in-patient, mental health services, and prescription drug coverage. The government has virtually no role in the direct delivery of healthcare which is administered by the sickness funds. The services covered under SHI are:

- In-patient and out-patient hospital services and care;
- Physician services;
- Preventive services, including dental checkups, checkups for children, immunizations, chronic illness checkups, and disease screenings like cancer;
- Care for mental health;
- Dental care and services;
- Physical therapy;
- Optometry services and care;
- Prescription drugs except for those explicitly excluded by law such as lifestyle drugs, including appetite suppressants, and those excluded because of a negative risk–benefit assessment;
- Medical aids and devices;
- Rehabilitation services;
- Hospice and palliative care;
- Maternity care and services;
- Sick leave compensation;
- Long-term care services and benefits.

This broad framework for SHI benefits is defined by law; however, specifics are determined by the Federal Joint Committee. Private benefit packages purchased by higher-income earners who opt out of SHI may be more extensive.

Sickness funds are financed by employers and workers through general wage contributions of about 14% and a contribution of 1% of wages, on average. The wage contributions are pooled nationally in a health fund called *Gesundheitsfonds* and are then reallocated to individual sickness funds. A risk-adjusted capitation formula is used, accounting for age, sex, and morbidity adjusted for 80 serious and chronic illnesses. In addition to compulsory wage contributions, the 1% supplementary, income-dependent contribution is paid directly to the sickness funds, the rate of which is determined by the fund. The unemployed contribute to SHI in proportion to their unemployment entitlements. The government covers the contribution for the long-term unemployed as well as providing copayment limits.

There are a range of deductibles in the sickness funds which require copayments for pharmaceuticals and in-patient services. Most deductibles and copays are in the areas of nursing homes, pharmaceuticals, and medical aids. Copayments are determined by federal legislation and apply at the national level. Citizens earning more than $68,000 can opt out and choose private health insurance instead. There are no government subsidies for private insurance. Unlike those in many other countries, sickness funds and private health insurers, as well as long-term care insurers, use the same providers. In other words, regardless of whether they are covered by SHI or private insurance, physicians and hospitals provide services for all patients. Civil servants are exempt from SHI; their private insurance costs are partly refunded by their employer. Military members, police, and other public-sector employees are covered under small programs that are separate from SHI.

About 88% of the population receives primary coverage through sickness funds, and 11% through private insurance. There are about 110 sickness funds in the country.

The federal government has wide-ranging regulatory power over healthcare but is not directly involved in care delivery. The Federal Joint Committee, supervised by the Federal Ministry of Health, determines the services to be covered by sickness funds. These determinations are based on evidence from comparative-effectiveness reviews and risk/benefit health technology assessments. The Federal Joint Committee also sets quality measures for providers and regulates the number of SHI-contracted physicians practicing. This is done using needs-based population/physician ratios.

The German healthcare system shares decision-making powers among the federal and state governments and self-regulated organizations of payers and providers. The Federal Joint Committee has 13 voting members: five representatives from associations of sickness funds, five from associations of providers, and three unaffiliated members. Five patient representatives have an advisory role but no vote.

A key point is that the government has the responsibility and control over setting prices. The Federal Association of Sickness Funds works with the Federal Association of Statutory Health Insurance Physicians and the German Hospital Federation to develop the ambulatory care fee schedule for sickness funds and the diagnosis-related group (DRG) rates, which are then adopted by bilateral joint committees. Germany's state governments also play an important administrative role. The 16 state governments determine hospital capacity and finance hospital investments and also supervise public health services. Regional associations of SHI-contracted physicians are required by law to guarantee the local availability of ambulatory services for all specialties in urban and rural areas. These regional associations also negotiate ambulatory physicians' fee schedules with sickness funds.

Private health insurance accounts for about 10% of total health expenditures. This consists of coverage purchased by individuals who can opt out of SHI, mostly higher-income individuals, those who are exempt from SHI, and supplementary coverage in policies bought by sickness fund enrollees. In 2017, 8.75 million people were covered through substitutive private health insurance. And in June 2018, there were 41 substitutive private health insurance companies in Germany.

Private insurance premiums are determined by individual risk evaluation, unlike in the United States where premiums tend to be risk related by groups with separate pooling charges. There are separate premiums for dependents. Risk is assessed only at time of coverage, with contracts based on lifetime underwriting. Younger people with good incomes find private health insurance especially attractive because as a result of risk-based premiums, insurers offer them contracts with a more extensive range of services and lower premiums. Private insurance represents supplementary coverage to SHI for sickness fund enrollees. Examples are covering some copayments for dental care and private hospital rooms.

The government plays a strong controlling role in private health insurance. It is regulated by the Ministry of Health and the Federal Financial Supervisory Authority to prevent the insured from being exposed to large premium increases as they age and are not overburdened by premiums if their income decreases. And the federal government determines provider fees under substitutive, complementary, and supplementary private insurance through a fee schedule. These fees tend to be higher than SHI fees. Preventive services do not count toward the deductible, and there are no copayments for recommended preventive services. There are no government subsidies for private insurance.

Sickness funds offer a range of deductibles and no-claims bonuses in their effort to compete for patients. Physicians who contract with sickness funds are not allowed to charge above the fee schedule for services in the SHI benefit catalog. However, a list of individual health services outside the comprehensive range of coverage may be offered for a fee to patients paying out-of-pocket.

Physician education is provided mainly in about 35 public universities offering degrees in medicine where tuition is free. The minimum qualifications for a medical degree are determined at the federal level by the Licensing Regulations for Physicians, state laws, and individual university requirements. Specialization requirements are regulated and enforced by the medical boards within each state.

Primary care doctors and specialists in ambulatory care typically work in their own private practices – around 56% in solo practice and 33% in group type practices. About 11% of physicians work in multiple specialty clinics and most of these physicians are salaried employees. Some specialized out-patient care is provided by hospital specialists, including treatment of rare, severe, or progressive diseases as well as highly specialized procedures. Typically, physicians employ medical assistants.

Individuals have free choice to choose among general practitioners and specialists. Registration with a family physician is not required, and general practitioners have no formal gatekeeping function. However, sickness funds are required to offer members the option of enrolling in a family physician care model, which has been shown to provide better services than traditional care approaches and often provides incentives for complying with gatekeeping rules.

Under SHI, general practitioners and specialists are reimbursed on a fee-for-service basis according to a uniform fee schedule that is negotiated between sickness funds and regional associations of physicians. The law requires SHI-contracted ambulatory physicians to be members of these regional associations, which act as financial intermediaries between physicians and sickness funds and are responsible for coordinating care requirements within their region.

Copayments or payments for services not included in the SHI benefit package are paid directly to the provider. In cases of private health insurance, patients pay up front and submit claims to the insurance company for reimbursement.

Physician payments are limited to a predefined quarterly maximum number of patients per practice and reimbursement points per patient, therefore setting quarterly thresholds for the number of patients and of treatments per patient for which a physician can be reimbursed. If physicians exceed the quarterly thresholds, they are paid considerably less for any additional services provided. This can lead physicians to postpone non-urgent patient visits once they reach the thresholds, which means patients may have longer appointment wait times at the end of each quarter.

For private patients, general practitioners and specialists are also paid on a fee-for-service basis. Private fees are usually higher than the fees in the SHI fee schedule.

As for hospitals, public hospitals make up about half of all beds, while private not-for-profits account for about a third. All hospitals are staffed principally by salaried physicians. Physicians in hospitals are typically not allowed to treat out-patients, but exceptions are made if required care cannot be provided by office-based specialists. Senior doctors can treat privately insured patients on a fee-for-service basis. Hospitals can also provide certain highly specialized services on an out-patient basis.

In-patient care is paid per admission through a system of DRGs, which are revised annually. Currently, there are around 1,300 DRG categories. DRGs cover all services and all physician costs. Highly specialized and expensive services like chemotherapy, as well as new technologies, can be reimbursed through supplementary fees. Acute psychiatric in-patient care is provided largely by psychiatric wards in general (acute) hospitals. The number of hospitals providing care only for patients with psychiatric and/or neurological illnesses is low.

Statutory LTCI is mandatory. The same insurers that provide SHI provide statutory LTCI. Employees share the contribution rate of 3% of gross salary with their employers; people without children pay an additional 0.25%.

There are many systems in place that ensure quality of care and better coordination of care and these are constantly reviewed for areas of improvement.

Reference List

1 Canada's Health Care System, Government of Canada, https://www.canada.ca/en/health-canada/services/health-care-system/reports-publications/health-care-system/canada.html.
2 Five Myths about Canadian Health Care, The Truth May Surprise You about International Health Care, by Aaron E. Carroll, Apr 16, 2012, AARP-Politics and Society, https://www.aarp.org/politics-society/government-elections/info-03-2012/myths-canada-health-care.html.
3 Podcast-Commonwealth Fund, https://www.commonwealthfund.org/publications/podcast/2018/oct/truth-about-waiting-see-doctor-canada.
4 New Poll Shows Canadians Overwhelmingly Support Public Health Care, Healthcare Now, Canadian Healthcare Coalition, Aug 2019, https://www.healthcare-now.org/blog/new-poll-shows-canadians-overwhelmingly-support-public-health-care/.
5 Healthy Canadians: A Federal Report on Comparable Health Indicators 2008, Government of Canada, https://www.canada.ca/en/health-canada/services/health-care-system/reports-publications/health-care-system/healthy-canadians-federal-report-comparable-health-indicators-2008.html, and New poll shows Canadians overwhelmingly support public health care, PNHP New poll shows Canadians overwhelmingly support public health care, PNHP Newsletter, Aug 12, 2019 http://www.pnhp.org/news/2009/august/new_poll_shows_canad.php.
6 Prescription Drug Coverage in Canada: A Review of the Economic, Policy and Political Considerations for Universal Pharmacare, by Jaden Brandt and Brenna Shearer, *Journal of Pharmaceutical Policy and Practice*, 11, 28, Dec 2018. Doi: 10.1186/s40545-018-0154-x, https://www.researchgate.net/publication/328790182_Prescription_drug_coverage_in_Canada_a_review_of_the_economic_policy_and_political_considerations_for_universal_pharmacare.
7 The Grass Is the Same Colour, Part II: Prescription Drug Woes on Both Sides of the US-Canada Border, by Oliver Kim, Health Affairs, Feb 13, 2020, https://www.healthaffairs.org/do/10.1377/hblog20200206.377829/full/.
8 Canadian Panel Calls for Universal Public Drug Coverage, by Kelsey Johnson and Allison Martell, *Reuters, Health and Pharma*, June 12, 2019. 11:52 AM, https://www.reuters.com/article/us-canada-pharmaceuticals/canadian-panel-calls-for-universal-public-drug-coverage-idUSKCN1TD20M.
9 International Health Care Systems Profiles, by Miriam Blümel and Reinhard Busse, Department of Health Care Management, Technische Universität Berlin, The Commonwealth Fund, June 5, 2020, https://www.commonwealthfund.org/international-health-policy-center/countries/germany.

Index

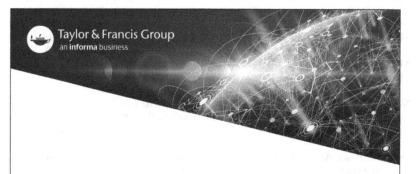